Your Irresistible Life

*4 Seasons of Self-Care through
Ayurveda and Yoga Practices that Work*

Madhuri Phillips and Glynnis Osher
Foreword by Maya Tiwari

BALBOA
PRESS
A DIVISION OF HAY HOUSE

Copyright © 2013 Madhuri Phillips and Glynnis Osher.

All rights reserved. No part of this book may be used or reproduced by any means, graphic, electronic, or mechanical, including photocopying, recording, taping or by any information storage retrieval system without the written permission of the publisher except in the case of brief quotations embodied in critical articles and reviews.

Balboa Press books may be ordered through booksellers or by contacting:

Balboa Press
A Division of Hay House
1663 Liberty Drive
Bloomington, IN 47403
www.balboapress.com
1-(877) 407-4847

Front and back cover photos: Michael Julian Berz
Artwork, Illustrations by Ryan Majeau
Layout and design by Glynnis Osher

Because of the dynamic nature of the Internet, any web addresses or links contained in this book may have changed since publication and may no longer be valid. The views expressed in this work are solely those of the author and do not necessarily reflect the views of the publisher, and the publisher hereby disclaims any responsibility for them.

The author of this book does not dispense medical advice or prescribe the use of any technique as a form of treatment for physical, emotional, or medical problems without the advice of a physician, either directly or indirectly. The intent of the author is only to offer information of a general nature to help you in your quest for emotional and spiritual well-being. In the event you use any of the information in this book for yourself, which is your constitutional right, the author and the publisher assume no responsibility for your actions.

Printed in the United States of America.

ISBN: 978-1-4525-7757-9 (sc)
ISBN: 978-1-4525-7756-2 (e)

Library of Congress Control Number: 2013912448

Balboa Press rev. date: 08/20/2013

Praise for *Your Irresistible Life*

"Simple, straightforward and enjoyable, Your Irresistible Life *is a wealth of practical guidance that can lead you toward good health. Even if you apply only a small number of the teachings and methods given here, you will discover the essence of Ayurvedic wisdom. How? Because you will feel better, and that increased vitality and wellbeing will reflect the higher level of self-knowledge that you have gained. Ayurveda is infinitely deep and profound, but its beauty and wisdom are within easy reach of everyone; this manual of practices can open the door to a direct understanding of this ancient tradition's compassionate healing power."*

~ David Crow, L.Ac.
Author, *In Search of the Medicine Buddha*

"It is always a pleasure to see good work arise out of sincere experience and experimentation. Madhuri and Glynnis have learned and used practical tools to reform themselves, and provided this accessible and valuable aid to help us do the same. Here's to a beautiful revolution of self-reformation!"

~ Dr. Claudia Welch, author of
Balance Your Hormones, Balance Your Life: Achieving Optimal Health and Wellness through Ayurveda, Chinese Medicine, and Western Science

"Madhuri and Glynnis have united the timeless wisdom of Ayurveda and the ancient spiritual discipline of Yoga in a most simple, practical way that can heal every individual and unfold the inner harmony of life in daily living."

~ Vasant Lad, B.A.M.S., M.A.Sc, Ayurvedic Physician
Author of *Ayurveda: Science of Self-Healing*, *Textbook of Ayurveda* series and more

"Instead of feeling exhausted at the end of each day, Your Irresistible Life *allows us to flow with the seasons, with the current of nature, finishing each day with the same energy as we started."*

~ Dr. John Douillard DC, LifeSpa.com

"With their earned expertise, Glynnis & Madhuri have made the immense power of Ayurveda so incredibly easy to practice—daily and deeply. As a big fan of Ayurveda, this is the system I've been looking for—both logical and loving, ritualistic and practical, ancient and modern."

~ Danielle LaPorte, creator of *The Desire Map* & *The Fire Starter Sessions*

"I dedicate this book to Ellen Msimanga."

~ Glynnis

"I dedicate this book to Jenny McLean Noble."

~ Madhuri

Contents

Acknowledgements xiii
Foreword by Maya Tiwari xv
Introduction xix

Part 1 Now We Begin

Chapter 1 How to Use This Book: Preparing for Your Journey 3
Chapter 2 I Intend 6

Part 2 The Essentials

Chapter 3   Ayurveda: It Doesn't Have to Be Complicated 11
Chapter 4   *Dinacharya/Ritucharya* (Daily and Seasonal Routine) 20
Chapter 5   Seasonal Food Practices: The Food Fantastic 26
Chapter 6   Self-Care Is Sexy Not Selfish 33
Chapter 7   The Truth About Yoga 36
Chapter 8   Breath Is Life: *Pranayama* Practice 41
Chapter 9   Meditation: "Is the Noise in My Head Bothering You?" 43
Chapter 10 Seasonal Ceremony and Ritual 45
Chapter 11 Cleansing: When? Why? How? 47

Part 3 Spring Time

Chapter 12 The Verve of Spring 53
Chapter 13 Spring Routines 59
Chapter 14 Spring Food Practices 61
Chapter 15 Spring Self-Care 69
Chapter 16 Spring Yoga, *Pranayama,* and Meditation 76
Chapter 17 Spring Ceremony and Ritual 84
Chapter 18 15-Day Sensational Spring Cleanse 87

Part 4 Summer Time

Chapter 19 The Exuberance of Summer 93
Chapter 20 Summer Routines 97
Chapter 21 Summer Food Practices 100
Chapter 22 Summer Self-Care Practices 109
Chapter 23 Summer Yoga, *Pranayama,* and Meditation Practices 116

| Chapter 24 | Summer Ceremony and Ritual | 124 |
| Chapter 25 | 7-Day Easy Juicy Summer Cleanse | 127 |

Part 5 Fall Time

Chapter 26	The Abundance of Fall	133
Chapter 27	Fall Routines	137
Chapter 28	Fall Food Practices	139
Chapter 29	Fall Self-Care	148
Chapter 30	Fall Yoga, *Pranayama*, and Meditation Practices	154
Chapter 31	Fall Ceremony and Ritual	163
Chapter 32	Fantastic 14-Day Fall Cleanse	167

Part 6 Winter Time

Chapter 33	The Hush of Winter	173
Chapter 34	Winter Routines	177
Chapter 35	Winter Food Practices	180
Chapter 36	Winter Self-Care	188
Chapter 37	Winter Yoga, *Pranayama*, and Meditation Practices	195
Chapter 38	Winter Ceremony and Ritual	204
Chapter 39	Winter Restoration: *Rasayana*	207

Part 7 Going Deeper

Chapter 40	Weird Ayurvedic Practices . . . That Work!	213
Chapter 41	Ayurvedic Home Remedies	215
Chapter 42	Tongue and Face Diagnosis	223
Chapter 43	Not So Common, Common Sense Ayurvedic Tips	228

Epilogue	231
Glossary	233
Bibliography	237
Resources	239
Index	241
About the Authors	245

List of Tables and Illustrations

Ayurvedic Doshas	14
Dosha Qualities	15
Determining your Dosha	18
Six Tastes and the Doshas	29
The Six Tastes: Their Actions, Elements, and Sources	30
Spring Food Guide	63
Spring Egg Mandala	86
Spring Cleanse Daily Check-In	90
Summer Food Guide	102
Summer Sun	125
Summer Cleanse Daily Check-In	130
Fall Food Guide	142
Nasagra Mudra	159
Fall Gratitude Tree	165
Fall Cleanse Daily Check-In	170
Winter Food Guide	182
I Ching	205
Winter Rejuvenation Daily Check-In	209
Tongue Diagnosis	225
Seasonal Tongue Diagnosis	226
Face Diagnosis	227

Acknowledgements

M

I would like to thank, acknowledge, and offer my love and gratitude to all of those who have supported me on my journey . . .

My amazing family; Shirley, Peter, and Richard who have always believed in me even when I jumped out of planes, shaved my head, and traveled around the world by myself with a backpack (countless times).

To Alistair, who without you, my life and this book would not be the same. Thank you for finding me again.

G

I give my deepest love and gratitude to my family, friends and all my teachers who have watched and supported, guided and encouraged, coaxed and comforted me through all of my on track and off-the-beaten-track choices and pursuits in my life.

My thanks and love to my incredibly spirited and creative family; my mother Minnie, my sister Debbie and my brother Shaun, and my nephews and nieces: Gregg, Dijon, Ava and Ella.

To my beloved husband Dave, you are my medicine buddha, my love and my greatest champion. I am so grateful and such a lucky girl to have you as my partner in this life.

G & M

As always we are inspired by and grateful to the Divine and Her cosmic sense of humour and timing in our lives. We are ever grateful to our teachers on this journey.

Our deepest thanks to all of the incredible souls who have helped bring this book into manifest form: Alistair Stewart, Dave Anderson, Karen Armand, Anna Busch, Mukulikaa Ananda, Gwen Nagano, Lalitadevi Tamburri, and Gail Taylor.

We are most honoured and give special thanks to Maya Tiwari for her loving acknowledgement of our journey and her profoundly insightful foreword.

Foreword by Maya Tiwari

In 1981, I introduced the first school for Ayurveda in North America. In those years, only the clinical protocols of Ayurveda had survived the ravages of time and misguided interests bequeathed upon this powerful science of health for humanity. Following my recovery from ovarian cancer, I explored the Motherland of India, hoping to find a school that had kept alive the *sadhana*—grassroots education of Ayurveda—the origins of the *Rishis'* vision whose cosmic mind informs that healing is neither prescriptive nor clinical. To my chagrin, no such school had survived the incursions of time. The original wisdom of Ayurveda supports each one of us to make firm the innate power to self-healing once we are in sync with the cyclical, rhythmic heart of Mother Nature. Through the Wise Earth School of Ayurveda, I took to restoring this ancient method for living—the way of *sadhana*—inner medicine healing. This education teaches us to mine our own extraordinary resource of inner medicine by living everyday in *sadhana*, preserving inner harmony and world peace. In re-establishing the ancient wisdom and ways of cyclical rhythms—daily, seasonal, lunar, and solar, we learn to awaken the memory and intelligence for absolute self-healing and profound peace. According to the *Atharva Veda*, Ayurveda's timeless education of *sadhana* is the most effective spiritual path to awaken consciousness and enhance our inner medicine potential for self-healing.

We are now ensconced in the central space of our world's authentic history—an incredible period of time when each and every human being can recover their inherent knowledge of the universe's cosmic rhythm, memory and *karma*. Poised in fullness of sentiency, we can relearn the ways of positivity—to act in kindness, and healing so that our response to life's grace and challenges transmute into a gentler, kinder self that brims with compassion. In this way, we learn to live simply and in reverence to all beings. Simply put, cultivating inner awareness is the way to reclaim our connection to Love, Light and Harmony for the benefit of all of humanity.

Glynnis and Madhuri's book adds to the light-bearers who carry the torch for humanity's wellness and healing. Through their long years of personal practice and sharing of this illuminating work, they have birthed a beautiful child, rich and simple in its integration of the basics of nature. Once we adhere to nature's cycles, seasons, breath, food, and sound, we become Whole-filled with the sentiency that gives *prana* to every grain of sand, each and every being in the way of harmony and goodness.

As you hold this precious tome in your hands, may you feel the healing vibration of manifold layers of wisdom and healing carried from the central womb of the cosmos to your heart.

Lovingly,
Maya Tiwari
Wise Earth School of Ayurveda
www.wiseearth.com

*"People travel to wonder
at the height of the mountains,
at the huge waves of the seas,
at the long course of the rivers,
at the vast compass of the ocean,
at the circular motion of the stars,*

and yet

*they pass by themselves
without wondering."*

~ St. Augustine

Introduction

Our Ayurvedic Adventure

Madhuri's Story

In the beginning, there was nothing. Nothing to be done—or said—just energy. This energy transformed into form and *taaa-da!* We have a manifested world with iPhones, talking robots, Botox, and high heels that surely weren't designed to walk in.

Amongst all of these material possessions, we are individual souls having a unique experience, learning and evolving through our life lessons here on planet Earth. Often, I forget this. Often, I get caught up worrying about paying bills or how my life will unfold or what to do next. Often, I forget the fact that *we are* Divine beings of great power and there are infinite possibilities in the magical creation called Life.

Years ago, just at the end of completing my four-year contemporary dance degree at Simon Fraser University, I had both an injury and then a strange growth erupt on my leg, leaving me only to hobble, not walk very well, let alone dance.

For the first time in my life, I was confronted with a self that did not know how to be happy being stalled, limping and not dancing. Not knowing who I was if I was not . . . The Dancer. My identity was intertwined with what I did, not resilient enough to endure the storms I was about to pass through. I felt like I was being punished, that God did not want me to dance or do what I really wanted to do more than anything in the world. Cue a heightened continuation of my spiritual journey and yet another new awakening.

This time proved to be the breaking open of my awareness to let in the light . . . and also a period in which I found myself jousting with the dark. For a decade, I was challenged with various strange illnesses and diseases that many medical professionals could not diagnose. I traveled back and forth between Canada and a number of other temporary homes—New Zealand, India, England. I found my Guru (although I was never looking for one), became a yoga teacher, got married, owned a yoga studio (which drained me both financially and emotionally), and began to study Ayurveda.

Luckily, my strength of character, tenacity, and curiosity forced me to pursue answers to my body's symptoms that doctors did not seem to know. I knew there had to be something on this Earth that could heal me so I took matters into my own hands. After studying Ayurveda, I integrated its principles, treatments, and modalities of healing into my own life, and began to heal myself.

Ayurveda works. Ayurveda helps us understand our own unique make up of the five elements and how we can balance our inner and outer natures. Doctors, therapists, shamans, yoga teachers—no one can heal us. It is Nature Herself that is the healer, and ourselves.

Ayurveda is a transformative process that harmoniously integrates body, mind, and consciousness. We cannot separate these aspects of ourselves if we are seeking profound healing and transformation. I found this out the hard way with many bumps along my path that I now see as gifts that carved out the direction of my life's purpose.

Part of my purpose is to share with you this beautiful healing art and science—Ayurveda—so that you may be empowered with the wisdom of Her and incorporate this spiritual medicinal philosophy into your life to balance, heal, and live the most healthy and joyous life you can live.

Many blessings on your journey,
Madhuri

Glynnis's Story

I was introduced to the mystical healing arts at a very young age. Growing up in South Africa, I had a nanny who was like a second mother to me. Her name was Ellen Msimanga and she was a *sangoma*, or Zulu witchdoctor and high priestess in the Zionist Church. Ellen would welcome patients to her small room situated in the back yard of our house. This was apartheid South Africa and there were many imbalances in the nature of things.

Ellen was a powerful healer and a loving presence in my life. I remember at night the scent of frankincense and the mysterious chanting of healing mantras sung in her native tongue, drifting out of her room, and soothing the turbulence of my heart. Those scents, sounds, and memories watered the seeds of my healing journey.

When I left South Africa at 23 years old to live in New York City, apart from the uprooting of my entire world as I had known it, a few key events moved to change the direction of my life towards an Ayurvedic healing journey.

I began a committed yoga practice, which kept me fit, both mentally and emotionally, for living a life in NYC. Here, I was introduced to Deepak Chopra's first book, *The Way of the Rishis*. This was the riveting story of his shift from traditional western medicine back to his Ayurvedic roots. I was utterly hooked and a loud YES! resounded through my entire being, waking up every sleeping part of me.

The second was my "unintentional" diversion in the form of my career as an art director. My background had been in graphic design and art direction, and upon moving to the United States I needed a sponsor for my green card if I was to stay. I was introduced to the owner of an advertising agency who was willing to sponsor me, but the catch was they primarily serviced pharmaceutical accounts.

I understood then, as I do now, the integration and importance of certain life-saving drugs for emergency medicine. I was appalled at the behind-the-scenes look at the evolution, marketing, and sales of these and other "wonder drugs". I was as troubled by other disturbing aspects of pharmaceuticals, namely their long-term detrimental effects on the planet, on our wellness as human beings, and our reliance on them as a society. I was working 15-hour days promoting an industry to which I mostly had an aversion. It made me heartsick. I longed for change and a way to connect my creativity to something more meaningful.

The third life-changing event was meeting Maya Tiwari (Mother Maya), Vedic monk and founder of The Wise Earth School of Ayurveda in North Carolina. The Food Sadhana course I took at the school introduced me to spices, chanting, mantras, Ayurvedic healing foods and breathing practices as I had never learned them before. I felt completely at home.

My soul was singing, shouting, celebrating, and remembering what it felt like to be connected to true beauty and grace though the awakening of cognitive memory. My given spiritual name from Mother Maya was *Prabha*, meaning "light, radiance, glow, shine, light-maker." Mother Maya described it as the dawn's first light. Indeed, it was as if a light had turned on in my life, which was to change my direction and propel me more deeply on the path of Ayurveda and to a deeper understanding of my true purpose in this incarnation.

Now almost 15 years later, having navigated through and explored within this vast and magnificent healing art, I am ready and excited to take this Ayurvedic journey through the seasons with you. I wish for us all, the pleasure of ultimate health, beauty, and grace. I believe a mindful and committed Ayurvedic practice is a sure road to an irresistible life.

Fragrant blessings of love and peace,
Glynnis

Part 1

Now We Begin

Chapter 1

How to Use This Book: Preparing for Your Journey

Our intention with this book is to guide you through a year long process that will radically transform your life to whatever degree you would like. We decided to live, explore, and enact the teachings of this book as we wrote it, putting ourselves through everything we are asking you to try out (and sharing with you some of our personal journal entries through the year).

Nature Herself will be your guide as she takes you through the changing seasons. We, feeding off Her wisdom and the proven solutions of Ayurveda and Yoga, will suggest a variety of appropriate foods, practices, and processes that compliment the time of the year. Each season is different from the next, so that what is beneficial during one season may not be optimal during another.

Align yourself with Her. Honor Her. Allow your own inner wisdom to be your greatest teacher. Your personal life will be the raw canvas of inspiration, challenge, and transformation. So please, begin this book at whatever season you choose.

Join us on this amazing journey as we introduce you to the ancient principles and practices of Ayurveda and Yoga, combined with our modern day sensibilities and savvy.

Everything in this book is here because it has helped us in our lives. We hope this book will be a strong, loving, and compassionate guide.

Wherever you may be, and wherever you would like to go, this book sets out to help you create the life you know you are here to live.

> "Spring passes and one remembers one's innocence.
> Summer passes and one remembers one's exuberance.
> Autumn passes and one remembers one's reverence.
> Winter passes and one remembers one's perseverance."
>
> ~ Yoko Ono

Paving the Way

Going on any journey requires some preparation, sorting out what to bring and what not to take, a clear direction, and an idea about what kind of journey you are taking.

The journey inwards is no different.

Here are some questions for you to journal to help you establish where you are, where you want to go, and how you are going to get there.

1. How do you define yourself?

2. What three things are most out of balance in your life right now or need the most attention? (Relationship, health, finances, career, creativity, family, fun, etc.)

3. What do you need to let go of to be more of the person you want to be?

4. What qualities do you need to cultivate or expand to be more of the person you truly are?

5. To whom or where do you give your power away?

6. Why do you give your power away?

7. What three things can you start to do today to live in alignment with the truth of who you are?

8. What would your ideal, non-negotiable self-care time look like?

9. What does making a commitment to your own self-care mean to you?

10. What is one thing you are willing to eliminate from your daily routine that is not serving you?

11. What is one thing you would be excited about incorporating into your daily routine?

12. a. What five words do you use in your day-to-day conversations that you would like to eliminate?

    b. And what five words do you rarely use that you want to use more often?

Preparation For Your Journey

The journey to your irresistible life begins now.

Preparing for your journey is about setting the foundation for your practice and helps you to begin with stability, confidence, and ease.

Having all the right tools sets you up for success in your commitment to your own self-care. We can often be stopped in our tracks if we suddenly find we are missing a basic support tool, or we do not plan properly for the journey ahead.

What You Should Pack for Your Journey

- Your intention.
- A journal to write your daily inspirations, affirmations, and observations.
- A yoga mat.
- A comfortable meditation pillow or chair.
- An altar space set up with your symbol of empowerment that can inspire and ground you.

First, Clear the Clutter

Where there is no space, nothing new will bloom. Think of the areas of your life that feel cluttered, full, or perhaps overflowing.

Is your to-do list endless?

Are your closets stuffed with things you no longer remember are there?

Is your mind overwhelmed with thoughts or beliefs that leave you in a negative mind-rut?

Clearing the clutter in all aspects of your life is essential in order to remove anything that is weighing you down, keeping you in an old version of yourself or one that you wish to evolve beyond.

Go through your closets and give away, recycle, get rid of the things you no longer need, use, or like. As you shift who you are, your beliefs, priorities, and energetic frequency will change, as will your preferences. Just let go!

Easier said then done. We understand. If you have a challenging time letting go of things start with smaller stuff like clearing out your bathroom and dispose of make-up or products that are aged or rancid. Clear your kitchen of old spices, herbs, teas, and foods that are well past their due date.

A fresh start.

Chapter 2

I Intend

Where the mind goes energy flows. Where you place your energy through thought, intention, and emotion will determine what you manifest in your life. If you are constantly focusing on the negative, you will see more of that. If you choose to see the positive and focus there, you will get more of the positive showing up for you.

Living intentionally is one of the most power-packed tools you can use to align yourself with the flow of life you wish to be in. Initially, this takes great practice, and eventually, it becomes so ingrained that you will be consciously co-creating your world and meeting life's ups and downs with greater ease and grace.

How to Set Your Intention

1. Phrase your intention in the positive.
2. Keep it fairly short and succinct so that it is easily repeatable.
3. Once you have chosen an intention that resonates with you, stick with it until it becomes manifest.
4. Write your intention out 50 times and repeat it as often as possible (sticky notes on the fridge, in your car, and on the bathroom mirror work as great reminders).

Setting your intention and energizing it daily is imperative to keeping you on track. Repeating your intention with heart and soul begins to reprogram the neuro-network that sends signals from your brain to the rest of your body.

You are what you think.

Most of what goes through our minds are thoughts, beliefs, or conditioning from our past. We react from circumstances or past experiences, very rarely from an empowered place of the present. The past is merely a story we repetitively tell. The present is creation. To live in the here and now, we need to be present and consciously see, feel, and know when we are choosing with awareness . . . or just reacting. This may be a lifelong practice as you continually refine your present moment awareness.

Sharing Our Personal Intentions From the Time We Spent Living and Writing this Book

M

My intention for the year is self-acceptance, self-love, and expressing myself creatively by being a clear channel through which the Divine energy can effortlessly flow. I plan to commit to my intention in the various aspects of my life in the following ways:

- *Health—experience increased vitality and balance through my yoga practice, biking, kayaking, and getting out into Nature.*
- *Wealth and Abundance—experience my true value and self-worth, and be well compensated for the work that I do in the world.*
- *Creativity—write a book!*
- *Fun—get back into dancing and spend more time with friends and family.*

G

I intend to thoroughly investigate the root causes of suffering in some areas of my life that are obstacles towards healing so that my spirit can flourish and I may fulfill my destiny.

- *I intend to commit to a life of beauty and joy through a steady self-care practice.*
- *I intend to walk this journey mindfully, transforming habits that no longer serve me.*
- *I intend to embrace a life of abundance, wealth, beauty, creativity, grace, and awareness.*
- *I intend to offer authentic service to others.*
- *I intend to play, dance, sing, create, shine, and love.*
- *I intend to give myself enough space and time to do this.*

Symbol of Personal Empowerment

Your intention is one tool for you on your journey. Your empowerment symbol is another way to connect with the energy of the direction you are choosing to go.

This symbol is the sign post for your journey to remind you that you are on track and to assist you to stay the course when obstacles, issues, and challenges stand in your way. Having a tangible symbol that you connect and resonate with is very powerful to keep you on the path and remind you of your strong intention.

Take some time to listen to your intuition rather than logically choosing something as your personal empowerment symbol.

Go out in nature or sit very quietly and ask yourself what symbol, representation, or object would most reflect your intention at this time. There is no right or wrong way to choose your symbol. Feel free to draw, paint, or colour it. Create your symbol, find it, and make it your own, whatever it is.

Once you are sure of your symbol, write down what it means to you and how it empowers you.

Sharing Our Symbols of Empowerment

M

My symbol of empowerment is a statue of Nataraj, *the Lord of the Dance. To me this statue represents power, vitality, and the ability to move gracefully with the flow of life.*

G

My symbol of empowerment is the Lotus. A Lotus flower symbolizes the sun, creation, and rebirth. At night, the flower closes and sinks under the muddy water. At dawn, it rises and opens again, growing into the light. To me, this flower represents the chance to begin anew each day without being discouraged by guilt and regret, or being bogged down by any shadows within myself.

Part 2

The Essentials

Chapter 3

Ayurveda: It Doesn't Have to Be Complicated

Ayurveda is derived from two roots: *Ayu*, meaning life; and *Veda*, which means knowledge. The knowledge of life, the science of life, is Ayurveda. Today, we associate Ayurveda with India and it can get confusing because some people think they have to eat Indian food or wear traditional Indian clothing to practice Ayurveda. Not so.

Ayurveda is an inclusive healing modality. It is the mother of all medicine, and, at its essence, it understands everything through the lens of the five elements theory. In India, this art and science has been developed, notated, and systemized for over 5,000 years.

The profound transformational practices within the scope of Ayurvedic Medicine are still being used today because they work, irrespective of culture or belief system. However, throughout time, every ancient culture and civilization embodied an understanding of living in harmony with nature: This organic evolution is how Ayurveda also originated.

- By observing Nature, we realize we are Nature: We are not separate.

- The five elements—earth, water, fire, air, and ether—make up everything on this planet, including you and I.

- We are all beautiful expressions of a unique alchemical combination of these five elements in distinct form. No two people have the exact same ratio of earth, water, fire, air, and ether.

When you learn the principles of Ayurveda, you will see how timeless and applicable they are to every single being. You will be empowered by connecting to the qualitative embodiment of how the five elements are not some esoteric idea, but a practical and applicable system to understanding how you can be balanced and healthy. This universal knowledge will be your greatest ally throughout your life as your health and needs continue to change. Awareness is the key to healing.

We must first be aware that we are not living in balance before we are inspired to make a change. So often it takes a major trauma or sickness before we are literally forced to reassess the way that we have been living our life. Sometimes, this comes in the form of an accident or disease; sometimes, it may be a divorce or loss of a loved one that wakes us up to the realization that we are not living the life we really want to be living.

Sharing A Realization of My Life Out of Balance

For me, it was an illness that the Western medical world was not able to diagnose or even treat that catapulted me into fully absorbing the practices and philosophy of Ayurveda. On one of my pilgrimages to India, I became very ill. A plethora of symptoms (fever, vomiting, diarrhea, delirious behaviour, sweating, coughing, and extreme fatigue) left me lying on a wooden bed at the ashram, wishing I were anywhere but there. I pushed through the illness, feeling guilty for not contributing to duties and chores, doing 16 hours of karma *yoga per day.*

After leaving the ashram, I continued on my planned journey, traveling through South-East Asia for seven months. It was not until I returned home to Canada that I was able to admit that I wasn't well. Previously, I was able to dance eight hours a day, but after my journey through Asia, just walking up a flight of stairs was exhausting.

I was sent by my family doctor to a foreign disease specialist in Toronto where every test known to man was conducted for all manner of illness: diabetes, parasites, AIDS, hepatitis, and on and on. I gave more blood than I thought I had and became really good at peeing into tiny plastic containers. After months of patiently waiting for my appointment with the specialist, I anticipated receiving a definitive diagnosis of my condition and a suitably great action plan. Nope.

I was told there was nothing wrong with me.

But, but, but . . . I wanted to scream. Cry. Give up. How could the specialist tell me there was nothing wrong with me when my body was clearly sick, exhausted, and depleted of all energy? I moved home to live at my Dad's place. I didn't have energy to hold down a job, let alone teach Yoga to anyone.

I knew there had to be something on this planet that could help. I set out to take my healing into my own hands. Enter Ayurveda. My healing was a process: It was not a quick overnight recovery, but through understanding my constitution and its imbalance, I was able to eat the proper foods, take the right herbs, and create a daily routine that had stable, lasting effects.

Ayurveda is now seamlessly incorporated into my life: It is not something I "do". It is the innate way that I live in accordance with nature by aligning with the seasons, times of day, and by knowing myself enough to adjust my thoughts or actions to prevent the accumulation of disease in my mind or body.

Prevention is always preferred over waiting until a full-blown disease erupts.

Disease does not happen overnight. It is often a process that happens over time with many subtle (or not so subtle) signals that the body, mind, or emotions have been trying to communicate, but we do not want to hear.

We want discomfort to go away, and yet, it does not. Over time, the knock at our door gets louder until we cannot ignore the steam train that just crashed through our living room with the horn screaming—*Pay Attention!*

Life wants us to pay attention, to learn the lessons we came here to learn and to be the best human being we can possibly be. This book was not written to help you get a better job, re-paint the bedroom, or wear more stylish clothes: This book was written to assist in connecting you to the deep calling from your soul that is asking you to wake up to the beauty and power that you are. You are a being of infinite potential who is sometimes trapped in fearful conditioning from society, your family, and your past.

Living in accordance with Nature takes us out of our comfort zone and into a fluid rhythm unique to us. Sound good?

Well, the transition from where we are to where we want to be, can, at times, be challenging. It leaves us oscillating on the threshold between who we have been and who we want to be. We must consciously choose and then take action, walk through the doorway, down the hallway, and into the garden of our life.

On this journey, you will need a guide who has tread the path to warn you about possible obstacles and to hold the torch to them as you take each step. We all have that light within us: We also benefit from having an external light in the world to assist us on our journey.

Let this book guide you as the deep, textured unfolding of your body, mind, and heart expand into a state of balance, ease, and grace.

Welcome to your Ayurvedic experience—a philosophy that is as ancient as human kind, delivered to you in a form that your mind, body, and schedule can digest.

Ayurveda 101

Ayurvedic principles stem from the basic understanding that everything is comprised of the five elements in varying degrees, so therefore, everyone and everything is unique. It is because we are all inimitable, we must understand what foods, lifestyle, and environment will be most supportive to us as an individual.

Your distinctive make-up is called your *dosha*, or constitution. Your *dosha* is an expression of your physical, mental, emotional, and energetic make up. At the moment of conception, your true nature is established: It is the blueprint, the ratio of the five elements that make up your *dosha*. Your true nature is called *prakruti.*

It is important to understand your *prakruti* to balance your self in a way to feel your best, to be healthy and happy. However, throughout your life you will go out of balance. Sometimes, a life's imbalance can begin in the womb if the mother is drinking alcohol, doing drugs, or is subjected to a trauma or stress.

Other times, the imbalance begins early on in childhood, as many parents do not understand Ayurvedic principles about how each child requires different care. Poor food choices for the individual, trauma, stress, moving, or even climate can begin to have an adverse effect that years later may manifest as a full-blown illness.

Into our teenage and adult years, the propensity for imbalance to occur accelerates as stress increases. Sometimes, we are simply trying to keep it all together in our life, with no time or energy to pay attention to the details of eating and living in accordance with our *dosha*.

The off-kilter state, however subtle or gross, is called, *vikruti.* The task of Ayurveda is to assist us in making the journey from our current state of imbalance—*vikruti*—back to our true nature (*prakruti*), where health is restored.

The five elements make up the three *doshas*: *vata*, *pitta*, and *kapha*.

The Ayurvedic *Doshas*

Vata = Air + Ether	Pitta = Fire + Water	Kapha = Earth + Water
Responsible for movement	Responsible for metabolism	Responsible for lubrication and structure
Primary location: colon	Primary location: small intestine	Primary locations: upper half of the stomach, chest

Let us now look at the five elements and see how they reveal to us the qualities that make up our psychobiological structure/constitution, or *dosha*. The elements have the following qualities:

EARTH: heavy, solid, dense, thick, dry, cold, rough, static, hard, stable

WATER: fluid, cold, moist, soft, smooth, heavy

FIRE: hot, sharp, clear, dry, light, subtle, mobile, penetrating

AIR: mobile, cold, dry, light, clear, rough, sharp, hard, subtle

ETHER: clear, light, dry, cold, mobile, sharp, subtle

Ayurveda is a qualitative science, as opposed to the Western model of quantifying everything. Understanding the qualities of food, thoughts, the time of year, and even the disease, makes it clear about how to achieve balance. The opposite qualities will be the ones that restore homeostasis.

Dosha Qualities

Vata Qualities	Qualities to Balance	Pitta Qualities	Qualities to Balance	Kapha Qualities	Qualities to Balance
Dry	Oily	Oily	Dry	Heavy	Light
Light	Heavy	Penetrating	Superficial	Slow	Fast
Cold	Hot	Hot	Cold	Cold	Hot
Rough	Soft	Light	Heavy	Oily	Dry
Subtle	Gross	Mobile	Still	Dense	Clear
Mobile	Still	Liquid	Dense	Soft	Sharp
Clear	Cloudy	Sharp	Soft	Static	Mobile

One basic principle of Ayurveda is that like increases like . . . and opposites reduce.

When we understand this, then all we need to do is simply look to the qualities of certain symptoms to understand how to come back to balance by welcoming in the opposite attributes.

For example, let us take the case of "Angry Angela" who has heartburn and acne. These symptoms are both of *pitta* nature: hot, inflamed, oily, sharp and intense. For Angry Angela to soothe her heartburn and acne, she would need to incorporate cooling foods (such as cilantro, basmati rice, mint, pomegranate, bitter leafy greens, and cucumber) into her diet. She could also increase her participation in cooling, non-competitive activities (like swimming, walks in the moonlight, laughing with friends, *pitta*-pacifying yoga). Most importantly, she needs to look at the mental and emotional aspects of underlying *pitta* emotions, such as anger, intensity, judgment, and perfectionism.

Each *dosha* has a balanced expression and an imbalanced expression.

No one *dosha* is better than the other, they all have their strengths and weaknesses. Even though we may be predominant in one or two of the *doshas*, we are made up of all five elements and, thus, all have earth, water, fire, air, and ether in different ratios to make up our individual unique self.

This means that *you* are perfectly YOU.

***Vata* individuals in balance** are creative, insightful, intuitive, active, imaginative, vibrant, and spontaneous due to the qualities of air and ether.

When out of balance, *vata* types may exhibit anxiety, nervousness, worry, insomnia, constipation, dry skin, bloating, gas, hyper-activity, fatigue, underweight, restlessness, muscle spasms, joint aches, intolerance of cold, low back pain, and an inability to handle stress.

To balance *vata*: follow a *vata*-pacifying diet; stay warm; drink warm fluids; eat cooked, slightly spiced, grounding/nourishing foods; avoid stimulants like alcohol and caffeine; self-massage with sesame oil; have a routine for eating, sleeping, waking; do not spend energy you don't have; do a gentle yoga practice, and practice *nadi shodhana pranayama* (that you will learn in the Fall Section).

Be particularly attuned to the *vata* practice in the Fall and early Winter season.

***Pitta* individuals in balance** are focused, ambitious, compassionate, bright, dynamic, vibrant, and make great leaders.

When out of balance, *pitta* types may act out with anger, aggression, manipulation, judgment, impatience, rashes, heartburn, fever, diarrhea, excess body heat, excess discharge of sweat, hot flashes, acne, visual problems, halitosis, acid stomach, and any "itis"—colitis, liver issues, and burn out.

To balance *pitta*: follow a *pitta*-pacifying diet; stay cool; avoid competitive sports and focus on less goal-oriented forms of exercise or fun; avoid the hot sun in the middle of the day; relax in nature; eat when you feel hungry; and practice *sheetali pranayama* (that is taught in the Summer Section).

Be particularly attuned to the *pitta* practice in the Summer season.

***Kapha* individuals in balance** are calm, nurturing, patient, reliable, consistent, stable, loving, serene, and have an excellent memory.

When out of balance, *kapha* types may be stubborn, passive, lethargic, apathetic, greedy, depressed, sleep excessively, or have slow digestion, swelling, upper respiratory congestion, obesity, nasal allergies, chills, or nausea.

To balance *kapha*: follow a *kapha*-pacifying diet; have ample spice in the diet; wake early; exercise daily; avoid over-eating; and practice *kapalabhati pranayama* (that can be found in the Spring Section).

Be particularly attuned to the *kapha* practice in the Late Winter, early Spring season.

What's Your *Dosha*, Darling?

Go through the following checklist twice.

To establish your *prakruti* (essential nature/constitution from the time of conception), initially check the boxes that relate to your long-term tendencies, or the way that things have been most of your life.

The second time through, check the boxes that relate to your *vikruti* (current state).

The checklist is merely a guide. Its accuracy is determined by the objectiveness of the individual. It is best to see an Ayurvedic consultant or practitioner to get a clear and accurate assessment of both your *prakruti* and *vikruti*.

Determining Your Dosha

	Vata	Pitta	Kapha
Physical frame	Slight, thin	Medium	Stocky, large
Body weight	Low	Medium	Overweight, dense
Eyes	Small, dry, active	Medium, deep set	Large, moist
Nose	Thin, crooked, bony	Medium, may have pointed tip	Short, round, thick
Skin	Cold, dry, rough, thin	Rosy, warm, oily, freckled, fair	Soft, thick, moist
Lips	Thin, small, dry	Medium, red, soft	Thick, smooth, oily
Hair	Dry, brittle, thin, fine, curly	Moderate, soft, often red, early grey	Thick, wavy, oily, lustrous
Face shape	Small, angular, long, asymmetrical	Heart-shaped, medium size	Round, large
Complexion	Rough, dry, tans easily	Rosy, prone to acne, oily	Pale, smooth, soft
Nails	Dry, thin, cracked	Soft, pink	Thick, firm, smooth
Appetite	Variable	Strong	Low
Digestion	Irregular, tends to have gas and bloating	Fast, tends to experience burning	Slow, tends to form mucus
Thirst	Variable	Excessive	Little
Elimination	Constipation, dry	Loose stools, burning	Thick, sluggish, mucus
Sleep	Light, tends to insomnia	Moderate	Deep, prolonged
Mental nature	Active, quick	Moderate, penetrating	Slow, steady
Emotional nature	*In balance*: flexible, creative, inspired, enthusiastic *Out of balance*: Anxiety, fear, stressed, confused	*In balance*: focused, joyful, confident *Out of balance*: Angry, irritable, impatient	*In balance*: calm, forgiving, patient *Out of balance*: Attached, greedy, stubborn, passive, apathy
Endurance	Low	Medium	Strong
Under stress	Overwhelm, anxiety	Rises to the challenge	Retreats, isolates
Likes	Creativity, travel, dance, movement, variety	Competitive sports, debates, intellectual stimulation, reading	Cooking, relaxing, dancing, music, gardening, nurturing
Total Prakruti (long term tendencies):			
Total Vikruti (current state):			

Once you establish your *prakruti* and *vikruti*, you can use the wisdom of Ayurveda to make conscious choices regarding food, lifestyle, yoga, exercise, career path, environment, and every other aspect of your life to maintain balance. These choices will help you have the energy to fulfill your highest potential.

Follow the guidelines in this book to help you understand how to bring seasonal balance through Ayurvedic practices, diet, yoga, meditation, and inner inquiry.

Most importantly, have fun and know that even doing a few of the suggested practices in this book will go a long way to enhancing your health and preventing nasty symptoms from rearing their heads and, thus, keeping you from your irresistible life!

Chapter 4

Dinacharya/Ritucharya (Daily and Seasonal Routine)

Everyday we wake up to new possibilities and opportunities.

Like a daily rebirth, we get to make or confirm choices, and take actions that can bring us great peace, calm, joy, and growth towards our self-realization. We are so blessed to have this day-by-day awakening; by living truly in the present with the perpetual gift of another chance, you allow yourself to build physical, mental, and spiritual health.

Daily practices are rituals of the most profound self-care and personal evolution, not a tedious and mundane regimen designed to make us rigid, obsessed, and dissatisfied. We must treat these daily rhythms as our sacred dance. They anchor, ground, and fortify us. They are our rock. They build character, awareness, and, through consistency, we see the fruits of our commitment.

We connect to our truth and we feel empowered.

All the practices provided in *Your Irresistible Life* will guide you through your day with compassion, companionship, and simplicity. You shall experience variations in your practices according to the changing seasons.

Each season, you will engage in specific practices that correspond with Nature's cycles and rhythms. These daily habits can bring harmony and order to your life, preparing the ground for illuminating your inner beauty and blessing your journey with grace and ease.

Mornings bring your first opening.

You could perhaps—if you do not already—attempt to arise at dawn (whatever time that may be wherever you are). As you gently brush off sleep, you feel every fiber of your body and greet each part of yourself with a gentle awareness, checking in before you get out of bed. You take a deep inhalation and stretch toes, feet, legs, torso, body, arms, hands, neck, and head.

Just before dawn, between 4 a.m. and 6 a.m., there is a special time where you experience a boon from the energy of the cosmos. This period is called *brahma muhurta*. This extraordinary time before sunrise offers a window in the pre-dawn hours that is most conducive for prayer and increasing your awareness.

As you are unburdened with worldly thought, this is a portal through which you can enter to offer your most sincere questions and receive greater clarity in response. You can benefit from this cosmic infusion even if you commit to waking with the morning birds only once a week.

You will see a shift over time, and an increased awareness in your daily life. This will mean setting your alarm for 4 a.m. Yikes! Try it just once and see if you notice any sparkling changes. All you have to do is show up.

Your Daily Routine

1. Your first step on arising is to scrape your tongue (preferably with a stainless steel scraper designed for this purpose), which gently removes the accumulation of toxins. This practice will assist digestion and eliminate bad breath.

2. Next, drink a cup of warm water. The water assists with evacuating the bowels and also helps clear toxins and unwanted accumulations in the body.

3. Swishing sesame oil around the mouth and teeth prevents bacteria from forming and can prevent gingivitis or gum disease. This is called oil pulling, and can keep gums and teeth healthy and strong, avoiding unwanted extra trips to the dentist or, even worse, extraction and/or loss of your pearly whites. The basic action is to push and pull the oil through your teeth and around gums until the oil becomes thin (about 10-15 minutes) and then spit it out into hot running water so as not to clog your drains.

4. You are now ready for some gentle yoga or exercise as guided by the seasonal practices laid out in each section.

5. *Pranayama*—breathing practice. This is nectar that becomes ever sweeter, the deeper into your practice you delve with dedication and consistency. Each season has a recommended practice.

6. Your morning, pre-bathing, *abhyanga* (self-massage) ritual—incorporating warm oils such as sesame, coconut, or sunflower—nourishes you. To heat your oils, place the bottle in a bowl of hot water until they are warm. *Snehana* is the Sanskrit word for oleation/application of oil. This word also means, "invitation to love and tenderness." As you massage yourself from head to toe, you receive the love of your practice. This brings suppleness to your skin and strength to your bones, among many other health benefits. Your emotions are nurtured, enhancing feelings of self-confidence, love, and awareness. Ladies, it is not recommended to practice *abhyanga* on the heavy days of your menstrual cycle.

7. A warm shower or bath washes away the oil leaving a fine trace to protect and lubricate the skin.

8. Now, engage in a morning face care ritual. Follow the practices for each season in the self-care chapters.

9. It is time then for meditation. Quiet your mind. Allow yourself the time, even if it is only 10 minutes a day, to connect and commune with the source that guides your intuition.

10. Breakfast offers your first opportunity to choose a meal that is aligned with your hunger and the season.

    If you are hungry, prepare a suitable meal and if you are not hungry, do not eat. This applies to all meals and gives you the opportunity to truly observe your digestion, hunger, and the needs of your body. It is wise, as part of the daily practice, to eat meals at a regular time each day. Avoid over-eating and gobbling down your food. Chew mindfully.

    Be diligent about making sure your meals are planned in advance as much as possible to avoid spur-of-the-moment choices that will not serve you. Don't settle for a less than ideal meal due to not making time for meal planning. It does no good for short—or long-term digestion.

11. Eating lunch between the hours of noon and 2 p.m. is the prime time for good digestion, so ideally try to make this the biggest meal of the day.

12. Afternoon, pick-me-up. Around 3:30 p.m. is a good time for one of the following: an afternoon elixir, a small snack, a piece of fruit eaten alone, a veggie mineral broth, and/or a herbal tea to keep you happy until dinnertime.

13. Dinner should be eaten at least three hours before bedtime to ensure ideal digestion, a good sleep, and rejuvenation of the body. How can you rest when your body is trying to digest?

14. Your evening practice may consist of: meditation, reading, journaling, reflection, art, and/or poetry. Activities that are not active! We strongly suggest you quiet the mind and turn off all electronic devices at least an hour before bed.

Sweet dreams and awake refreshed for a new day!

Daily practice is also about choosing a livelihood that fits who you are and not only supports you, but also brings you joy and satisfaction.

When your cup is full of joy and abundance, you have freedom to rest, relax, restore, and offer service to others. This is the real reason for organizing your day and observing your daily practice. Bringing order through daily ritual affords us more of the rare commodity of our era—more time.

Where there is no chaos there is no stress. Where there is no stress, there is space for play, community, family, and being available and fully present in every moment for yourself and others.

One-Day Wonder Day

"What a difference a day makes..."

Is it not true that one day of stressful deadlines, a sick child, or a fight with a loved one can really take it out of you?

Conversely, a day dedicated entirely to the soul purpose of pausing, re-connecting, and providing deep nourishment to yourself is exactly what the One-Day Wonder Day is all about. If you are too busy to do this at least once a season... well, you're too busy!

Take a day out from your regular responsibilities to bask in the silence and quietude within yourself, or to re-evaluate what adjustments need to be made in your life to be more aligned with your own nature.

Prevention

It often takes a major life event or trauma for us to pay attention to what is going on in our lives. By being aware of how you are feeling about your career, relationships, your health, and yourself, and by staying connected to the rhythms of life, it becomes very obvious when you are not in your flow. Have you ever felt that things are just not right? You know something needs to change, but you are not quite sure what it is or how to go about it?

Having this day to replenish and rejuvenate is a wonderful remedy to re-connect with what really matters in your life. Turn off your phone. Send the kids to the neighbour's place. Do what you have to do to make this happen. You are worth it!

What you will need for your day:

- A journal.
- Delicious, wholesome food (or you can stick solely to the Ayurvedic cleansing food, *kichari*—refer to seasonal *kichari* recipes in the Fall and Spring Recipes and Meal Ideas sections).
- Herbal teas of your choice.
- Epsom salts and essential oils for your bath (refer to essential oil recommendations in the Aromatherapy section for each season).
- Organic oil for your self-massage; cold-pressed sesame oil if your body needs warming and grounding; coconut oil if you need cooling; and sunflower oil if you need lightening up.

Your One-Day Wonder Day Schedule

Now, if you are like many people and have a daily to-do list and feel great satisfaction at checking off each item, you may think a transition day is a bit of a waste of time when there is so much to get done. Or perhaps you have spare time in your life but it's poured into doing things that you don't really want to be doing, like watching TV, or over-eating out of boredom and loneliness.

This One-Day Wonder Day schedule is a guideline only. Feel free to add or delete anything that doesn't mesh with you. However, watch the sneakiness of the mind if it's trying to get out of things that it doesn't like. Watch for excuses such as, "I'll skip the yoga bit because I'm not very flexible," or, "I'll just check my e-mails a few times throughout the day in case there is something really important that comes through."

The One-Day Wonder Day is meant to get you out of your habits and offer you a different experience.

Therefore, we highly recommend that you turn off all electrical devices for the day (phones, cell phones, TV, radio, and computer) to create space so that you have time completely to yourself for as much of the day as possible.

- Your One-Day Wonder Day begins the night before. What time you go to bed and the quality of sleep you have will completely influence how you feel the next day. Get to bed by 10:30 p.m. at the latest the night before to wake feeling refreshed and rejuvenated.

- Upon waking, set an intention for yourself, or simply repeat to yourself: "Today is a wonderful day!"

- Scrape your tongue.

- Self-massage—*abhyanga*—using the seasonally appropriate oils.

- Have a cup of warm water with a squeeze of lemon.

- Follow the seasonally appropriate yoga practice.

- Follow the seasonally appropriate meditation practice.

- Journal. Take three minutes to write whatever comes to mind. Do not lift your pen from the page; keep writing until the time is up. Don't over-think this exercise. Allow the stream of consciousness to flow through you even if none of it makes any sense.

- Breakfast: choose whole foods that are nourishing and satisfying for you and seasonally appropriate.

- Read, draw, write, dance, create a vision board, imagine, dream, play . . .

- Lunch preparation: Cook your lunch mindfully and be aware of your thoughts as you cook. Consciously infuse your food with love. We highly recommend the Ayurvedic superfood, *kichari*.

- Walk in Nature.

- Afternoon: relaxation, meditation, journaling, free time!

- Dinner: To give your digestive system a well-deserved rest, we recommend *kichari* for dinner, too.

- Gratitude journal: write down 20 things that you are grateful for in your life. As you write down each person, item, or experience, feel the qualities or essence of that which you are grateful for.

- Warm bath with 1/2 cup Epsom salts and three drops of lavender essential oil or appropriate essential oil for the season.

- Before bed: Massage warm oil into your feet and slip on some old cotton socks so your bed sheets don't get soiled.

- Set the intention to have a wonderful night's sleep: "I shall fall asleep quickly and easily, and I will wake feeling refreshed."

Chapter 5

Seasonal Food Practices: The Food Fantastic

"The doctor of the future will give no medicine but will interest their patients in the care of the human frame, in diet, and in the cause and prevention of disease."

~ Thomas Edison

We are made up of the sun (fire), rain (water), air, and soil (earth) within the container of space (ether). The components constitute the *Panchamahabutas*—The Five Great Elements.

The plants, through photosynthesis, garner these elements to bring life, vital nutrition, immunity, and growth. The animals, through eating the plants and also other animals, are in turn nourished through the same five elements. We are, in turn, nourished by the plants and the animals, and our waste returns again to the earth. The cycle continues in an ideally symbiotic relationship so that all of life is created, nourished, and grown to full potential and an ultimate state of glowing health. This continuous process of origination, succession, and renewal is life and food as it is meant to be.

Let us consider how true this is to our own personal food practices, and how we can get as close to this interconnected model as possible. Why? It is because food is about consciousness and not just about what we put into our mouths.

Food consciousness is about concerning ourselves with where our food comes from, where we choose to shop, how we prepare it, the way in which we eat it, the environment in which we eat, and the times of day we sit down to meals. Consciousness is about the mindfulness we have through the entire process of nourishing and sustaining ourselves.

G

I love and relish, with great passion, the preparation and enjoyment of food. My sister and I often contemplate whether our love of food comes from our Jewish roots, where major events always happened around an abundant feast. Perhaps our challenges with over-eating, emotional eating, and eating to soothe the soul also draws from this same ancestry where, throughout history, abundance of food or the deprivation thereof has played such a crucial role in defining a people. We wonder if it is settled deep within the DNA of our heritage. It is a big topic of conversation, humour, and tenderness with us. Food has the ability to make us feel deeply nourished and taken care of, or if we abuse it, to make us feel guilty, uncomfortable, and desperate.

My most transformative personal eating experiences have been in the mindful observances of the Earth-based practices learned and inspired by Mother Maya at The Wise Earth School of Ayurveda.

These are practices according to the cycles and seasons of Nature and of truly listening to what the body needs, beyond the habitual cravings—this is an Ayurvedic approach to food.

There have been times where, uninterrupted, I have observed with strict discipline a diet designed for my personal constitution according to the seasons. This is where I mindfully prepare all my meals, offer my gratitude before each meal, and eat slowly with appreciation for my food.

Leading up to a meal, I grind and meld my own masala spice blends, make my own weekly ghee *(clarified butter) as a meditation, and do not stray. I observe the correct food combining, eat with moderation, and eat only the foods that balance my* pitta/kapha *constitution. When I am determined not to waver from this path, my body transforms in 12 weeks. My skin becomes smooth, clear and glowing; my hair, shiny and strong; my body, agile and toned; my digestion, excellent; and my energy, vibrant.*

When I follow this disciplined path for a longer time, I feel both fantastic and also somewhat restricted. I have come to realize the need to allow for the free flowing flexibility of life and the satisfaction of occasional food desires and delicious treats. Otherwise, a part of me is miserable. The learning here is that the "perfect place" for our personal constitution followed too rigidly is not realistic for most of us as a lifestyle, nor is it sustainable.

Several years ago, I was diagnosed with three very large uterine fibroids, which a medical doctor suggested I have surgically removed. Instead, I followed a three-month focused and extremely disciplined Ayurvedic food practice as I described above. Along with the prescribed diet, I included a specific Ayurvedic herbal regimen created for my condition and constitution. I was doggedly determined, as I felt my life was at stake considering my family history of ovarian, breast, and other cancers. In three months, and to the disbelief of the Western medical community, an ultrasound showed my body had reduced three uterine fibroids of eight centimeters, six centimeters, four centimeters, all to zero, completely gone. I allowed my body's healing wisdom to perform its miracle. It took mindfulness, discipline, and a genuine desire to bring my body back into balance so I could make this happen. Prevention rather than cure.

There is a time for more stringent measures, more closely followed food regimens, but a balanced plan of daily conscious eating has longevity and gets you off the dieting mentality and into the space of positive habits that are sustainable for life.

> *Many of the practices I gained through my studies at The Wise Earth School of Ayurveda have stayed with me and are naturally woven into my daily life. It has taken me years to unfold and integrate these practices. They are still a work in progress as I peel off the layers of old habits, deep emotional traumas, and food challenges.*

We receive constant news in the world of food around calories, proteins, carbs, superfoods, vegetarianism, veganism, raw food lifestyles, etc. and we are somewhat overwhelmed and confused. What do we choose? How do we eat? What makes the most sense?

Simplicity and going back to basics is the answer:

- Fresh organic food less traveled.
- Moderate eating.
- Unrefined whole foods.
- Seasonal eating.
- Wild fish—not farmed.
- Grass-fed, farm-raised animal foods—not factory farmed.
- If you are vegetarian, the same goes for your veggies—alive, local, seasonal, and fresh.

By making these conscious choices, you are participating in the symbiotic, mutually respectful relationship of all life.

In Ayurveda, we also observe proper food combining for good digestion. Foods that are not compatible in the digestive system will eventually turn into toxins in our body and become the precursor to disease. There are various reasons that certain foods do not combine well: the post-digestive taste; the digestive acid required to digest certain foods; and the qualities and characteristics of certain foods.

It makes sense that certain foods do not go well together. However, people often see these combinations as normal and part of an everyday meal. Some examples would be: beans with cheese (as in burritos); eggs with a glass of milk; and fruit with milk (milkshakes). Fruit eaten with any other food is not a good combination (with the exception of cooking dried fruits such as raisins, berries, or apples into other foods). Keep things simple by eating fruit two hours before or after meals.

Sweet, Sour, Salty, Bitter, Pungent, and Astringent

In Ayurveda, we talk about the six tastes. There are major benefits to including all of them in every meal for optimal digestion, and for nourishing all of the tissue layers of the body. Each taste has a special and unique function and acts as a guide as to how to nourish ourselves so that we can avoid cravings and satisfy our nutritional needs.

As we move through this journey together, we will see that we literally are what we eat. We will look at the importance of the six tastes and how our digestion, absorption, and enjoyment of food are affected by feeding our body the tastes of sweet, sour, salty, bitter, pungent, and astringent. All foods have a primary taste and possess more than one taste, and therefore, offer multiple benefits to the body's nourishment.

These charts will help you understand the principles, actions, and sources of the six tastes and can be used as a guide when preparing meals.

The Six Tastes and the Doshas

Taste	Balances	Aggravates
Sweet	Vata and Pitta	Kapha
Sour	Vata	Pitta and Kapha
Salty	Vata	Pitta and Kapha
Bitter	Pitta and Kapha	Vata
Pungent	Kapha	Pitta and Vata
Astringent	Pitta and Kapha	Vata

The Six Tastes: Their Actions, Elements and Sources

Taste	Balances	Elements & Qualities	Sources
Sweet	Increases bulk and builds body tissues. Adds weight and moisture to body. Nourishes skin and hair. Sweetens voice. Soothes mucous membranes.	*Earth and Water:* heavy, moist, and cooling.	*Sweet fruits:* peaches, mangos, bananas. *Grains:* wheat, rice and barley. *Dairy:* ghee, butter, cream. *Sweet vegetables:* sweet potatoes, butternut-squash, yams, carrots, beets. *Sweeteners:* maple syrup, cane sugar. *Spices:* cinnamon and cardamom.
Sour	Cleanses tissues. Relieves thirst. Stimulates digestion. Assists in absorption of minerals. Sharpens the senses. Increases the appetite.	*Earth and Fire:* hot, light, and moist.	*Sour fruits:* lemons, grapefruits, and limes. *Fermented foods:* pickles, sauerkraut, and soy sauce. *Sour dairy:* yoghurt, buttermilk, yellow cheese, and sour cream.
Salty	Enhances the other tastes. Lubricates tissues. Maintains mineral balance in the body. Helps eliminate wastes.	*Fire and Water:* hot, heavy, and moist.	*Salty sea vegetables:* kelp and nori. Sea salt, rock salt. *Spices:* celery seed.
Bitter	Stimulates appetite. Detoxifies and cleanses tissues. Cleansing to the liver. Cools inflammation internally and externally.	*Air and Ether:* light, cool, and dry.	*Bitter green leafy vegetables and herbs:* kale, spinach, dandelion, basil, arugula, parsley, cilantro. *Bitter fruits:* bitter melon. *Bitter spices:* fenugreek, turmeric, cumin, fennel, coriander.
Pungent	Stimulates digestion. Expels and clears mucous. Promotes heat and sweating. Detoxifying. Aids in digestion, circulation, and enhances an active metabolism.	*Fire and Air:* hot, dry, and light.	*Hot and spicy foods and spices:* onions (raw), garlic, ginger, chili peppers, black pepper, cayenne.
Astringent	Reduces water due to absorptive action. Tightens and draws together issues. Cleanses and eliminates toxins. Heals wounds and ulcers. Dries out excess moisture and fats in the tissues. Purifies the blood.	*Air and Earth:* cool, dry, and heavy.	*Legumes:* most dry beans and lentils. *Fruits:* cranberries and pomegranates. *Vegetables:* asparagus, turnips, and broccoli. *Grains:* rye and quinoa. Coffee and tea. Aloe gel/juice. *Spices:* fenugreek, saffron, cumin, turmeric.

Romancing Your Relationship with Food

How would you describe your relationship with food?

Is it a love/hate relationship? Scarce? Indulgent? Full of guilt? Feast or famine? Passive-aggressive?

Food is something we cannot do without, so it is crucial that we make friends with our body, cravings, and ideas/beliefs around food. Ideas about food were instilled early on within all of us, depending on the household in which you were brought up. As children (and now as adults, if unresolved) eating times were more than just about food. Power struggles, striving for independence, and/or demanding personal choice were all tied into what and how we ate. We cannot stop eating; otherwise, we will literally perish.

We must make friends with food, our body image, and the way we relate to nourishment.

Our very first form of nourishment is (more often than not) the milk from our mother. It is not only nutrients that we receive from breastfeeding, but connection, bonding, warmth, and love, as a mother gives selflessly to sustain her young.

Food is nourishment, our connection to the Earth and to the Divine. When we eat with an attitude of gratitude, we actually absorb more of the nourishment, nutrients, and *prana* from the food. When we eat in a distracted or hurried state (while on the computer, talking too much, or without awareness), our digestion does not function as well as it does when we take the time to say a prayer or take a few deep breaths to slow down and be conscious of what we are putting into our body. What we ingest becomes our body and influences our mental and emotional states.

Here are a few tips to help you make lifelong friends with your food:

M

> *Be aware of what you are eating. Carry around a notebook for at least one week. Write down the time you eat, what you eat, and how you feel before and after you eat. During my Ayurvedic training, this was one of our assignments. I came to realize that I was always feeling irritated before I ate, and that I waited too long in between meals for my particular constitution. Once I saw this pattern, I was able to correct it, and now I always carry a bag of almonds with me just in case my blood sugar begins to slide.*

Say a prayer, grace, or take a few deep breaths before you eat. This practice is not religious (though it can be). This ritual is about creating an energetic connection to what is about to become you. We should be grateful for the amazing tastes, textures, and colours of food. It's incredible that we have access to an abundance of food day to day. Remember how blessed you are.

Slow down, chew your food, and eat in a calm environment. This is a large aspect of how well you digest. By chewing your food properly, (until it is a liquid pulp) you will pre-digest your food and increase the absorption in your small intestine. Eat in a relaxed environment. When the body is in a stressed state it does not give any energy to digestion as it is functioning in fight or flight mode.

Make eating sacred. This doesn't mean it has to be serious, but the more we honour our food and all of the people that contributed to us getting it (the farmers, the truck drivers transporting it, the grocery store clerk and on and on), the more we will respect our own body and lessen the tendency to over-eat or fall into unhealthy eating patterns. Eating becomes an experience of love and gratitude, an expression of thanks for life itself and an acknowledgement that we survive and thrive through our interdependence.

Food Prayer

Divine Mother, give us food, health,
and prosperity for the body,
efficiency for the mind,
and above all,
Thy love and wisdom for the soul.

Om. Peace. Amen.

~ Paramahansa Yogananda

On our journey we will look at practical and simple food guides through the seasons, how to choose your food and plan your meals, work with herbs, seeds and spices, explore simple and delicious seasonal recipes, and incorporate food rituals for fantastic health for your whole mind, body and spirit.

We embrace the empowering Ayurvedic principle that food truly is our medicine, and that good digestion is the gateway to the happiness, health and stability in our life.

To your health!

Chapter 6

Self-Care Is Sexy Not Selfish

Self Care is about Soul Care.

When we truly learn to love ourselves, we feel inspired to take care of our body, our mind, our daily practices, our work, our food, and our families. Not in the way where we sacrifice ourselves and our own well-being, but where we put ourselves first and express our undeniable truths. We deeply and truly take care to be all that we are—and we are solid. Do you love yourself? Close your eyes, take a deep breath, and look inside.

See beyond the physical structure, the self-appointed flaws, the bad hair day, the good skin day, the wrinkles, the frown, the ego, and/or the smile. Think about the way you take care of your soul. What is it you love to do that makes you feel beautiful beyond anything else . . . where, no matter what anyone says, you would not be knocked off your feet? What is that thing that makes you feel so deeply loved, confident, and taken care of that you can say without any doubt, "YES!" . . . I love myself?

Daily practices of conscious self-care—your *sadhana*—will cultivate and connect you to that love and innate self-appreciation, especially in those times when you are finding it hard. Daily connections with soul-affirming, joy-abounding, ego-blowing self-truths will remove all hesitations in answering this big important soul question.

G

From the ages of five to twelve years old, all I wanted to do was tap dance. I went to dance class three or four times a week and by the time I was eleven, I had completed all my tap exams with Honours with Distinction. *Every time I was on stage dancing, the exhilaration and joy I felt was unlike anything else I had experienced. I felt alive and good and happy and completely 100% okay. Better than great. I loved the costumes and the make-up and the music and mostly the unbelievable thrill of the sound and rhythm that came out of me and my tap shoes.*

In 1975, my last year in primary school, I was appearing in a dance film in South Africa called The Best of Everything. *I had a few duets and solos for which I was laying down the tap sound tracks in the studio. Most days there was an intense but glorious schedule of dancing from morning to night. I had stayed back from my beloved annual school trip in the* bushveld *(the South African countryside) so that I could continue to practice and be in the film. Those of us left behind who did not participate in the school trip were out on the field one afternoon doing gymnastics, an activity I also loved at that time. As I ran onto the springboard readying myself to fly over the vaulting horse, the springboard jammed and I came crashing down to meet it. I completely shattered my right hip, and also obliterated my dreams of a dancing career. I was completely off my leg and, for an entire year, had crutches to help me move around like a one-legged whirlwind. Even though the sound tracks for my dance roles were used in the film, I did not appear in it.*

I felt crushed, but, somehow, the joy I had within me was not.

I spent that year discovering other things about myself that I may not have paid attention to if I had not been forced to do so because of my accident. I realized I could write poetry and loved to express myself through that craft. My writing pulled me through a delicate and vulnerable time in my life.

As an adult, I recently went back to take a series of tap classes, and the moment I began to dance, that unfettered joy came flooding back to me and I smiled the biggest, most child-like, ridiculously carefree smile for the entire time I was taking the class. For whatever reason, that rhythmic tapping dance makes my soul soar and floods my body with pleasure hormones.

So now as I get deeper into what self-care means for a lifelong practice, I know it is many things . . .
- *Meditation*
- *Daily sunbaths*
- *Moonlight walks*
- *Concocting natural cosmetics*
- *Fresh whole food prepared with love and intention*
- *Listening to music*
- *Being in nature*
- *Yoga*
- *Painting*
- *Singing*
- *And, of course, dancing*

You name it. It is your joy to fulfill. Your self to care for.

Conscious self-care can be one or all of these things, done with love, intention, and joy. This is *sadhana*. Together we are going to explore the practices we love and those that will stick. What we have come to appreciate is the long-term rewards that come from consistency and that can be measured over time by good health and true joy of mind, body, and spirit.

In an Ayurvedic approach to self-care, there are daily beauty and soul-feeding rituals for each season that are designed to bring you glowing health and exquisite skin.

These are beauty routines that smooth off the rough edges of your life and bring out your radiance and inner confidence. We invite you to discover completely natural, easy-to-make beauty products straight from your home apothecary with the recipes offered in this book.

Self-care beauty routines and soul-care practices reflect the commitment you have to honouring your self and your life.

Chapter 7

The Truth About Yoga

What is Yoga?

Most people conjure up images of young, slight women in next to nothing contorting their bodies like it was a Cirque Du Soleil audition, or perhaps the stereotypical image of a peaceful looking person sitting out in nature somewhere in the cross-legged lotus position, eyes closed and index fingers touching thumbs.

M

My first foray into Yoga was unintentional. I had a dance injury and still wanted to move my body while I recovered. I quickly became more interested in the connection between the mind and Yoga, even more so than the physical aspect of the practice. I recognized at a young age that the body is susceptible to injury, illness, and decay, yet the mind is such an elusive and powerful beast. A beast I naively thought I could learn to tame and master by the age of 25.

A series of serendipitous events landed me in the poorest state of India at the Bihar School of Yoga, the world's first Yoga university. I had no idea about gurus and certainly wasn't going to bow down to anyone. Being a self-proclaimed atheist and feminist, I was sure I knew what I was doing and didn't need help from anyone else, thank you very much.

Like a moth to a flame, I entered ashram life as if it was as natural as the birth of a new day. I loved the simplicity and rigour of constant karma *yoga (selfless service) that consumed most of my time at the ashram. I found an odd satisfaction and pleasure cleaning the toilets before dawn, seeing the sunrise everyday for six months, and practicing periods of* mouna *(silence).*

One night after a prophetic dream, I awoke and set off to find the barber that would come to the ashram once a week to shave all of the swamis' heads. I sat down on the ground and signaled to him. He began to snip away my locks that kissed the middle of my back. Once there was enough of a clear-cut of the forest on my head, he went in skillfully with the blade and shaved my head to the scalp.

I was naked.

It took days for some people in the ashram to recognize me, and many of the Indians in my class thought I was nuts—a Western woman shaving her head?!

I took initiation with my Guru, received a personal mantra and was given my spiritual name, Madhuri, *meaning inner beauty, inner sweetness.*

As a lifelong over-achiever, I became the best li'l yogi out there, embracing karma yoga to the point of exhaustion and chanting my heart out every night at the evening kirtan *(call and response sing-song with tabla and harmonium).*

I was on the road to becoming a swami if only it wasn't for one thing . . . love. My beloved was back in Vancouver, and he was never out of my mind and heart. I was not destined to live out my days wearing orange pyjamas and renouncing everything in the material world: friends, family, boyfriend, and the adventures beyond the ashram walls. Despite always feeling like I had one foot in the world of the ancient Sanyassin tradition and one foot in my life outside, the inner shifts that I experienced during my time at the ashram were palpable and affected my life completely.

After leaving the ashram and re-integrating into my life, things started to crumble around me. I was not established in my self, but caught in two apparently conflicting lives that didn't have a merging point in sight. I lost my relationship and felt displaced for years. In earnest, I taught yoga, trying to convey to so many students over the years that the practice is much more than just sweating in downward-facing dog.

Now, 15 years later, I have come to realize that Yoga is not about wearing the latest yoga pants, nor is it necessarily renunciation and escaping our responsibilities in the world.

Yoga is an attitude . . . not just one you tap into as you move through your day, but, more importantly, a conscious approach you engage in as you move through your life.

Yoga is the way in which we think, act, and feel in our human experience.

Yoga is the expression of humanity that connects us to the Truth of who we are—Divine Beings of Spirit. We are all infinitely powerful creators. Unconsciously, we create struggle, pain, and illness. Consciously, we choose who we are and how we want to be in the world despite what curveballs life throws at us.

Yoga is not about being good . . . or holy . . . or righteous. Yoga is about unraveling all of the threads of the glorious tapestry of our life, laying it out, and saying, "YES!" When we say yes to all that we are and embrace the shadow that we neatly tuck away (so that no one will think the horrible things about us that we think about ourselves) this is the beginning. When we take complete and utter responsibility for our life and choose to abide in the richness and love of existence—these actions epitomize Yoga.

Once you take complete responsibility, my friend, you construct the framework and foundation of a pure Yoga attitude for any downward-facing dog you will ever do. Your practice should not be undertaken without awareness. Awareness is what makes any action Yoga. When we wake up and realize that we are not our parents, nor are we the conditioning of society, or who we were yesterday, we create ourselves anew from the present. When you operate in the present, there is freedom. There is freedom to choose who you want to be now. Allowing yourself this gift of transformation unleashes you from the constraints of the small life you were living and opens you up to a connection more powerful and beautiful than you could ever have created without aligning yourself to the Source of all that is.

The universe does not want us to struggle. The universe wants us to thrive.

We have certain lessons to learn before we can move to the next level of awareness, of Being. Often those lessons come as challenges that force us to confront the shadow that is so neglected.

M

I am always amazed to read yoga teachers bios that go on about how peaceful and heavenly Yoga has made them and that they claim to exist in a state of perpetual bliss. Really?

For me, Yoga has been the most challenging path.

It is a path of ruthlessness, tearing away what doesn't work to reveal who I need to be in the world. It is a never-ending path luring me forward and testing my discernment and strength of character and heart. The ground is not solid. It is in a constant state of flux, forcing me to find my centre, the part of me that is, in fact, unchanging.

So what does any of this have to do with what we know as Yoga here in the Western World? Everything. Your little rubber yoga mat is like a magnifying glass for what is going on in your mental and emotional bodies and boldly demonstrates how your thoughts are intrinsically connected to your physical body.

The physical aspect of Yoga is the tip of the iceberg, but let us not ignore the depth and immensity of what exists below the surface. The yoga *asanas* (postures) are designed to keep you healthy by benefiting all of the systems of the body. The nervous system, digestive system, circulatory system, reproductive system, and so on, are all strengthened when doing the specific practices appropriate for you.

Traditionally, Yoga was passed on one-on-one, from teacher to disciple. The student would take the disciplines, or practices, go and do them for a set period of time until they were perfected and ready to "advance" to the next level of awareness. A student may be given a *sadhana* or spiritual practice to perfect over a number of years before adding anything to it. In our fast-paced, goal-oriented society we want to know we are progressing or achieving when we are investing time into an activity.

Practice Yoga for the sake of practicing Yoga.

The benefits will come, no doubt, but do not focus on your achievements, as this is a trap and will lead to comparison and dissatisfaction.

The Ayurvedic approach to Yoga considers all aspects of who you are and what you need to support you in your life right now, taking into consideration: climate, age, level of health, as well as mental and emotional stress. Yoga is used to bring balance.

Therefore, the principle of "opposites reduce" is wise to follow. If you are feeling over-heated or agitated, you will need a cooling practice to balance yourself. If you are feeling overwhelmed, anxious, and stressed out, you will need a grounding, calming, and centering practice. If you are feeling dull and lethargic, then you will need a more dynamic and invigorating practice.

Each yoga posture is a well-designed instrument that has specific effects on the mind and body. In this book we have created sequences for you to practice which will allow you to create equilibrium within a specific season as we are all affected by what is going on in Nature—we are Nature.

Four Season Warm-Up

Learn this simple and quick warm up to move *prana* through the joints and loosen up any stiffness you may have in the body. You can do this anytime, anywhere, all year long before your seasonal yoga practice.

From a standing position:

1. Shoulder rotations (30 sec.):
    - Inhale, roll your shoulders forward and up towards your ears.
    - Exhale, roll your shoulders back and down.
    - Repeat 5X in the forward direction and 5X in the backward direction.

2. Neck Warm-up (30 sec.):
    - Exhale, lower your chin down towards your chest.
    - Inhale, roll your head to the right until your right ear is over your right shoulder.
    - Exhale, circle your chin back to the centre of the chest.
    - Inhale, roll your head to the left until your left ear is over your left shoulder.
    - Repeat 5X.

3. Hip Circles (30 sec.):
   - With your feet at least shoulder width apart and parallel, place your hands on your hips.
   - Move your pelvis in large circles 5X in one direction and 5X in the other direction.

4. Knee circles (30 sec.):
   - Bring your legs together.
   - Place your hands on your thighs just above your knees . . . bend your knees.
   - Move your knees in circles 5X in one direction and 5X in the other direction.

5. Ankle rotations (30 sec.):
   - Lift your right heel until your weight is up on the ball of your foot.
   - Circle your foot around the ankle joint while keeping the ball of the foot on the floor.
   - Move in one direction 5X and then rotate the ankle in the other direction.
   - Repeat with the left foot and ankle.

Chapter 8

Breath Is Life: *Pranayama* Practice

We arrive into this world on an inhalation and depart on an exhalation. In between, we take 20,000 breaths per day. We can live without food for 40 days, without water for four days, and without air for only a few minutes before life ceases.

The breath is the most essential aspect of life, yet how often are you aware of your breath? Luckily, we do not have to consciously command the body to take each breath in and out; otherwise, our whole life would be focused on survival.

The ancient *Rishis* and Yogis realized that the breath is intrinsically connected to the mind and body. The state of the breath is a doorway of insight into the mind and emotions. This becomes more obvious in stressful times where you find the breath is shallow and the chest tightens.

Conversely, in a relaxed and peaceful state, the breath is deep and easy.

The breath is the foundation of your Yoga practice.

During countless yoga classes anywhere in the world, at almost any time, students strain and force themselves into postures while jeopardizing their peace of mind and their breath. Without proper breathing, you are not practicing Yoga, no matter how complicated the pretzel-like position into which you twist yourself.

In order to have a powerful yoga practice (and life), you must understand the relationship the breath has to every cell, muscle, and organ in the body. The breath is your fuel, your guardian, your friend, and your lifeguard. The breath and the nervous system dance together to create a beautiful waltz—or a clumsy tap dance. When you take slow deep breaths you automatically communicate with the para-sympathetic nervous system to take charge and relax the whole body. Short, shallow breathing alerts the sympathetic nervous system that you are in danger and the fight-or-flight mode kicks in, compromising your system and draining you of vital life energy.

Your life energy is known as *prana*. You may have also heard this term described as *chi*, *qi*, or *ki*. It is your *prana* that carries the breath through the body, and it is your life force that animates you and provides you with more or less energy, depending how you take care of it. Stress and tension drain your life force, while conversely, balancing your schedule and filling it with creativity, joy, and harmonious relationships enhance your *pranic* energy, providing you with a strong energy field.

We have all had experiences of walking into a room or encountering a situation that felt heavy, sad, or perhaps even violent, and how this adversely affected our energy. Every thought, feeling, word, and emotion is energy and has a particular frequency. You also carry a certain frequency. Some days your frequency may be giving out joyful and welcoming vibrations, and some days you may be communicating a frequency that says, "Leave me alone."

Working consciously with the breath allows you to expand your *pranic* energy.

The Yogis devised a series of practices called *pranayama* to manipulate and expand the dimension of *prana*. You will be guided through various *pranayama* practices relating to the season as you move through the different chapters of this book. Daily *pranayama* practice will provide you with rich results as you use the breath as the bridge between the mind and body to consciously become the master of both.

Chapter 9

Meditation: "Is the Noise in My Head Bothering You?"

Meditation is not something that you do. It is a merging of consciousness and form. Closing your eyes and focusing on your breath is not meditation. Meditation is a merging of awareness of the meditator and the object of meditation. Uniting with the universal consciousness—The Mother, God, Spirit, whatever name you would like to give—is the state of meditation.

Even by talking about meditation we cannot understand, nor can we analyze meditation to get us any closer to the experience. This state, however, can be experienced in infinite ways. Some people connect through rock climbing, scuba diving, writing, dancing, looking at the ocean, or being with their child.

There is no right or wrong way to be.

M

> *I have spent years sitting down cross-legged on the floor, focusing on my breath, sometimes very agitated with my "monkey mind" jumping here, there, and everywhere; and sometimes slipping into a state of extreme peace and stillness, feeling the pulse of the universe.*
>
> *This is the practice of meditation. The biggest misconception about meditation practice is that it is bliss. Years ago, I went to a 10-day silent meditation retreat. Was I ecstatic, levitating, and communing with God? No, it was grueling. My knees hurt, my back ached, and I couldn't wait for meal times. What I did learn was how much my ego or personality wasted energy through mindless talk and habitual responses to people. I saw the juxtaposition between being silent and not looking at another human being for 10 days and how connected and loved I felt, opposed to being in the busy city seeing many people and feeling so alone.*

Sitting still, we are able to observe the tendencies and craziness of the mind and therefore gain some perspective that our thoughts are, in fact, separate from who we are.

But if we are not our thoughts or even our emotions, then who are we?

This is a question humans have been asking themselves since time immemorial and one that we must continue to ask.

Life feels so personal. Me—my—mine! We connect and cling to our thoughts and emotions as though they are real. Yet how can something be so real when it is constantly changing? If you are your thoughts then what were you thinking last Thursday at 2:15 p.m.?

Sitting down to meditate is using the tool of stilling the body along with a technique to train ourselves to let go of the strong attachments and identification with the idea of who we are, if only for a few minutes.

The gaps between thoughts are where the magic and beauty lie. Those are the moments we experience peace and safety as we are reminded that we are not alone as we struggle through life trying to survive. The universe does not want us to suffer. The universe wants us to wake up to the power, creativity, and joy that we are. The universe is constantly inviting us to remember that we are a soul in a body, floating in a sea of consciousness through this magnificent and mysterious expression of life.

Throughout this book, meditation practices will be provided to you. You are encouraged to try them consistently, everyday for at least 40 days in a row.

You do not need to take a lot of time in your day for meditation.

Even 5-10 minutes as a daily practice will have a profound effect on your physical, mental, and emotional well-being as well as the way you experience your life.

Chapter 10

Seasonal Ceremony and Ritual

The performing of ceremony or ritual in the Hindu tradition is known as *yagna* or *yajna*, and is usually a multi-layered and sometimes elaborate ritual of releasing or giving up prayers, offerings, or materials into a sacrificial fire. The Hindu *yagna* is an outer form of worship in which offerings are made to various gods and goddesses to purify and appease and to ensure various transformative outcomes. These ceremonies are accompanied by mantras, the chanting of various seed syllables and sacred verses from the Vedic texts. These rituals have become less practiced as they are looked upon by newer generations—who have moved away from the traditional ways—as complicated, empty, or foreign.

Still, there are many homes and temples where these rituals are performed for all kinds of occasions: births, deaths, weddings, graduations, and to bring prosperity. With the outer display of worship comes the inner practice. Ceremony and ritual create an action to be taken. A tantric approach to connecting with the higher self. A reminder and a physical connection to the elements, the soul, the source. An engagement with life on earth and a conduit to the world of spirit.

The inner practice is the deeper work that comes through that connection and seals into your personal life map the memory of meaning.

We perform ceremonies daily for various things. We make them up without realizing it. What if we created them with intention and used them as a tool to mark important times of transition, celebration, accomplishments, gateways, and gratitude. These ceremonies or rituals, when performed with awareness, are burned into limbic memory and awaken our cognitive memory so we can acknowledge where we are and progress on our path, move on from things that no longer serve, fit, or bring us love.

These rituals encourage us to grow, break free from old patterns, and begin anew.

They facilitate change.

Ceremony revives our participation in the dance of life as we experience it here on Earth. It is an intentional physical act of devotion for a specific outcome with the purpose of moving us forward.

G

A couple of years after I left South Africa and was living in New York City, my beloved Zulu nanny, Ellen Msimanga, died suddenly of a heart attack. I was grief-

> stricken as she had been like a second mother to me. I was also guilt-ridden, taking on the collective shame of white South Africans for the wrongdoings towards the black people in apartheid South Africa. I was left with many things unsaid, many questions unanswered, and I needed closure. By divine intervention, I met someone who directed me to a Nigerian witch doctor living in Harlem who he said could help me achieve this closure.
>
> Late one night, I made my way to his small room in an apartment on 128th Street and was greeted by an older man wearing traditional witch doctor's garb. We sat down and he proceeded to ask me questions. I told him all about Ellen and my struggles with letting go, and he advised me to let her rest, release her spirit to the spirit world, and stop holding on through my attachment, grief, and guilt. He threw some bones mixed with various other objects, a ritual I had seen Ellen perform before in her role as a sangoma (medicine woman). He chanted for a while and then stopped. Everything was quiet for a few minutes. He then said to complete this ritual I would need to bring him a live chicken to be sacrificed. I said I could not, and I left.
>
> Although I felt some connection to Ellen from this ritual, what I really got from this experience was that I needed to perform a ritual in the language of my own heart. I placed a picture of Ellen on a simple altar that I had created, lit a candle, and made a cup of black tea with boiled milk and sugar in a tin mug I had from South Africa—exactly the way Ellen used to make and drink it. I felt comforted as I sat gazing into the candle and sipping the warm, sweet tea, talking with Ellen's spirit, crying softly, and then falling into a deep sleep. I woke up feeling refreshed, and through this deceptively simple ritual, I felt as if I had said goodbye and could release her, forever keeping her love and memory in my heart.

Your own *yagna* or *yajna* practice should involve the following actions: create your space, your altar, your ritual, your ceremony to seal in and acknowledge these gateways of time and life experiences; celebrate and acknowledge with ceremonies that connect you in a solid way with sense memories to integrate and mark the passages of your inner and outer life.

Chapter 11

Cleansing: When? Why? How?

To cleanse or not to cleanse? That is the question.

The Ayurvedic perspective on cleansing is very unique and specific to the person, time of year, climate, constitution, and the state of health of the one who is cleansing (just like everything in Ayurveda).

We have certainly gone overboard in our society with our obsession to keep everything clean, at least on the outside. Time, energy, and money are spent on facials, manicures, new clothes, make-up, and body creams, yet how much time and focus do you allocate to thinking about the cleanliness of your insides?

Ayurvedic and yogic practices are designed to clean you from the inside out. You do not have to stand in a flowing river and draw water in through your anus, drink gallons of ghee, or swallow a piece of cloth to get benefits from a good, old-fashioned Ayurvedic cleanse.

The intention of this book is to offer you four various cleansing approaches to gently give your digestion a break, eliminate built-up *ama* (toxicity) in the mind and body, and build your *ojas* (vitality).

Each season offers you a different approach for supporting these processes while honouring how *vata*, *pitta*, and *kapha* manifest in our internal and external environments, depending on the time of the year.

Why Cleanse?

Pollution in the water, air, and soil leaves fruits and vegetables lacking the nutrients that our grandparents enjoyed. Only a couple of generations ago, all food was organic, animals were not fed hormones, and our carbon footprint was not even a concept. In the last 100 years, the quality of our food has diminished rapidly. Not only that, but our awareness around eating and the sacredness of breaking bread and coming together has been replaced with lunches on the go, family dinners reserved for major holidays, and watching "the tube" while scoffing down a plastic-wrapped microwavable delicacy.

Toxins and pollutants make it harder for the body to digest and assimilate what nutrients are left in the food, and when food is not digested, *ama* builds up in the body. *Ama* is a thick, heavy, sticky, mucous-like substance that clogs up the body and prevents it from functioning properly. When our body becomes full of *ama*, a myriad of symptoms may result such as fatigue, indigestion, gas, bloating, or constipation. When the digestive *agni* (fire) is weakened, *ama* begins to accumulate.

Given time and proper circumstances, this situation can be the ripe beginnings of what later may become a full-blown disease as the *ama* spills out from the digestive tract into the other *dhatus* (tissues of the body such as plasma, blood, muscle, adipose/fat, bone, nervous, and reproductive systems).

Once the body's channels become clogged, the proper flow of *prana* is disrupted, which sends *vata, pitta*, and *kapha* into frenzied states of confusion.

This stagnation of nutrients and absorption has an impact on the mind as well. Ah yes, the mind. It can also generate and be susceptible to *ama.*

Our thoughts may be the most toxic of toxins.

More toxic and deadly than a second piece of chocolate cake, more toxic than the DEET in your mosquito repellent, and even more toxic than smoking. Gasp! The mind is our most powerful friend or foe.

When we cleanse, we delve deeply into the arena of clearing out *ama* of both the mind and body, and thus it is important to have a few boxes of tissues at hand to allow those tears to flow if necessary.

How Gunk Accumulates

Ama accumulates from a poorly functioning digestive system or digestive fire due to:

- Eating fried foods, refined sugars, red meat, too much wheat, or heavy foods
- Processed, canned, or microwavable foods that lack *prana*
- Lack of exercise
- Consuming too much water with a meal
- Drinking ice cold drinks
- Environmental pollutants and toxins
- Eating without true hunger (emotional eating/eating out of boredom or obligation)
- Excessive alcohol
- Eating when emotionally distressed
- Stress

How to Get Rid of *Ama*

First and foremost, take a candid look at what and how you are eating, digesting, and eliminating. From there it's time to give your digestive system an overhaul. Specifically, observe whether you have any symptoms—such as gas, bloating, chest pains, stomach aches, or flatulence—after you eat. Do you have low energy, aches in your body, lack of concentration, or difficulty sleeping? These may all be signs pointing towards a buildup of *ama* in your mind and body.

By following the steps, tips, and recommendations in this book you will create small miracles for yourself. You will begin to reduce the buildup of toxicity that has accumulated from a number of factors you may not have even noticed: years of poor food choices which were not appropriate for your constitution; eating late; too much travel; and way too much stress.

All four of the seasonal cleanses in this book are designed for you. Follow them, do them, and live the results. Stay on top of your health day to day so you do not fall into a binge/cleanse rut (which is not healthy). And if you are serious about doing a deeeeeeeeep cleanse, find a reputable *Pancha Karma* centre that offers this ancient Ayurvedic treatment of restoring health on a profound cellular level.

One Size Does Not Fit All

The most important aspect of feeling healthier and thriving in your life is listening and honouring your own unique inner wisdom. This is easier said than done, granted. However, practice makes . . . practice. The more you learn in theory and then apply in your life, the more you will see that:

"Nothing is right for everyone and everything is right for someone."

This ancient Ayurvedic aphorism is the essence of what Ayurveda is all about. This is true for any of the information in this book. Please listen to what is right for you at any particular time. Honour that, and you will truly be practicing Ayurveda.

Timing is Everything

It is *not* always a good time to cleanse. Too much cleansing is not better. Looking honestly at your intention for cleansing is key to a healthy and successful cleanse. For example, "binge cleansing" is not sustainable or beneficial. A binge cleanse is when you eat or drink way too much and then flirt with an eating disorder. Under the guise of a cleanse, you restrict yourself from everything until the next time you go on a sugar, alcohol, or drug bender. Sound familiar?

Establishing a healthy relationship to your food and body, while keeping your insides clean and in good working order, is essential. In Ayurveda the change of seasons is the ideal time to cleanse. This helps to prevent the accumulation of *ama* and to prepare the body for the upcoming season. If you are taking care of yourself consistently and not allowing too much toxicity to build up in the first place, you will not need drastic measures to stay on top of things.

If you are going through a divorce, have recently lost a loved one, or are under enormous amounts of stress, these are not the times to cleanse. Make sure that when you embark on any form of cleansing that it is done in a way that honours yourself, your body, and what may surface for you as the mind sheds any debris that is ready to be released. You need to create the appropriate time and space in your life to graciously go through a cleanse.

Pancha Karma (five actions) is a traditional form of a deep cleanse where disturbed *doshas* are drawn from the *dhatus* (tissue layers), drawn back into your digestive tract where the disturbance originated, and then eliminated in various ways. *Pancha Karma* is a very intense and thorough cleanse that must be supervised by an experienced Ayurvedic practitioner and is not something to be taken lightly. In India, there are *Pancha Karma* hospitals where patients may spend months on a very simple diet, observing silence, and getting various daily treatments to overcome disease.

The cleanses in this book are designed so that they complement your busy modern life, while still giving you the opportunity for profound healing and transformation. You will reap the benefits of the cleanses when you take the time to schedule in rest and relaxation during these periods.

Part 3

Spring Time

… Chapter 12

The Verve of Spring

"There are only two ways to live your life. One is as though there are no miracles. The other is as though everything is a miracle."

~ Albert Einstein

Skipping in the sun, dodge ball at recess, dandelions, ducklings, and one step closer to Summer . . . it's Springtime! Time to breathe a sigh of relief as the days grow longer and the darkness of Winter fades to light.

Smiles appear on the faces of strangers passing by, buds erupt on the tree branches outside the windows. We don lighter jackets and stuff cumbersome winter coats to the back of the closet. Our chests feel open, and an air of positivity and possibility wells from inside, woken from Winter's hibernation. We want to move, to run, to ride a bike, and to just go.

Freedom.

Inner sensations are being reawakened. Our cells literally feel more alive. Fresh! There are colours bursting, blossoming rhododendrons kissing shoulders as we walk by, as inspiration returns in the form of an inner thirst to be outside with Nature.

Springtime is the *kapha* time of year. In this season, things thaw out, melt, liquefy, and soften. *Kapha* literally means overflowing water; however, out of balance *kapha* can be inert, lackluster, and weighty.

To keep *kapha's* tendency towards lethargy at bay, now is the time to move. Get out and shake it up!

Enjoy foods, sights, smells, and activities that are invigorating, energizing, and dynamic to help clear out excess mucous, toxicity, and stagnation that may have accumulated in your body throughout the Winter season.

You need only look to Nature to observe the opening, flowering, and expansion that occurs in the Springtime. This precise form of awakening is being mirrored within us in body, mind, and heart.

Having the courage to let go of stagnancy or anything that we have outgrown is essential to the re-birthing process. Perhaps there is a wardrobe, friendship, partnership, or job that is weighing us down, keeping us in an old perception of who we were, not who we are *now*.

Can you relate?

By now, we should have all learned through trial and error (a.k.a. life) that we must move forward and not ruminate over things that are not allowing us to be who we want to be. You are the one with the power to decide who you are now, how you are in the world, and how you want to show up and express yourself.

The more you stay in your flow and connected with Source (insert God, Creator, Nature etc.), the more you live from an authentic, empowered place that is less directed by the external and driven by your internal guidance.

This empowered place is freedom.

This flow can happen anytime you choose. In the Spring, however, is when you are flushed clean with the thawing of your heart's fears to step out and embrace the wholeness and fullness of who you are.

8 Spring Journal Questions

1. What does the Spring season represent to you?

2. What qualities are invoked within you during Spring?

3. What you love about the Springtime is . . . ?

4. What three things can you do for yourself this Spring to stay balanced physically, mentally, and emotionally?

5. Where would you like to direct your energy this season?

6. How can you make this happen?

7. What aspect of yourself is no longer serving you that you are ready to evolve out of?

8. What aspect of yourself would you like to expand?

G & M's Spring Journals

G

April 16th

In 1996, while traveling in India, I received a gift of a simple rosewood mala from a man who I believe was a holy messenger. One of those messengers who are sent by the divine when we are most lucky or most needing a nudge or reminder of something greater than our smaller less cosmic concerns. I met Surendra in Haridwar, near Rishikesh, as I was walking through the marketplace. He was a professor of music, and full of life wisdom. We had a wonderful time over those legendary cups of Indian Chai discussing Vedic astrology, sacred music, and other intriguing topics. After a rich afternoon of conversation, I mentioned to Surendra that I was leaving for Rishikesh the next day by train and we said our goodbyes. I was sitting waiting at the station the following day, and Surendra magically appeared on the platform just before my train was due to arrive. He walked slowly up to me, handed me a very simple dark rosewood mala and said to me in a deep and sincere voice, "meditate."

Then he walked away.

So extraordinary life is. As I was writing a story about the meaning of malas in my journal, I went to the kitchen to make a cup of tea and my treasured rosewood mala caught on the kitchen cabinet and broke.

They say when a mala breaks you are not supposed to fix it. You are supposed to gather it broken and place the beads on your altar, that it is time to move on and let them go because you have learned something, made a breakthrough. New lessons are ready to come your way in this university of life. Time to choose and connect with a new mala.

There is a part of me that wants to fix this mala and ignore the wisdom of letting go. It is the third one this year that has broken on me. The first one I was more attached to the beauty than the sentiment or energy of and so I let it go quickly. The second was a sandstone mala I had bought for my beloved as a gift, which I chose to wear one day as adornment. It was unthinking to wear someone else's mala. This, the third one, made me really quite sad. It was a special gift steeped in meaning, and given to me with a specific message in a city regarded as one of the seven holiest places to Hindus.

In Hindu mythology, Haridwar is one of four sites where drops of Amrit—*the elixir of immortality—accidentally spilled over while being carried in a pitcher by the celestial bird* Garuda*. The* Kumbha Mela, *a holy festival held every 12 years in Haridwar, attracts millions of pilgrims, devotees, and tourists. These seekers congregate here to perform ritualistic bathing on the banks of the river Ganges to wash away sins and attain Liberation.*

I have been wearing my rosewood prayer beads on and off over the last 16 years stopping now and then to think about the profound gift of them, and who they came from. Now those words "meditate" float in the ether around me. No beads imbued with a reminder of this practice that leads to immortality. The message seems more profound now especially as I have of late recommitted to deepen my practice.

To meditate, I do not need anything except for my desire to feel peace and communicate with the divine, with the source, with my own divinity. Surendra . . . thank you. Perhaps those difficult planets you mentioned that have been obstructing the course of discipline in my practice have also shifted, and the timing is perfect for the creation of something new to come into being. I am sure somehow this was all destined and 16 years was the exact life span intended for this most treasured mala.

M

*April 10*th

There is always a time in one's life when change must occur. Perhaps I'm a slow learner. Perhaps I am stubborn or self-righteous, or perhaps I am human, doing the best I can . . . I feel fairly balanced in many areas of my life; however, I am fully aware of how little play time and down time I have had in my life recently (ok, the last seven years).

I am fairly disciplined naturally. I like routine and I enjoy doing things that make me feel better. I have had a consistent yoga practice for over 17 years now, yet, I have to admit, I find it challenging to relax at home. Possibly because I work from home and my computer seems to have a vortex around it that sucks me in and draws the very life force out of me through constantly checking e-mails, doing bits and pieces of administrative work for my business and reminding me that if I don't check Facebook I might be missing out on some life threatening information . . .

So, I'm consciously taking steps towards my personal self-care, which involves spending more time in nature, with friends, and making sure that I laugh more (yesterday I bought Glynnis and I each a pair of funny and kind of creepy glasses with eyes in them. It's amazing how it really doesn't take that much to amuse me . . .).

Looking back to the earlier years of my life, and even up until university, I felt that joy was a predominant state for me. I'm not sure if it was the stress of feeling that all of a sudden after I graduated it was me in this big ol' world trying to survive, but an air of competition and trepidation crept up and nabbed me in the mind, knocking me out of my natural state.

The lovely combination of financial stress and ill health set me into a feeling of me-and-the-world, like we were on opposite teams playing British Bulldog. A game I never particularly enjoyed at the best of times.

Now, I am committed wholeheartedly to love myself no matter what. I have decided to do away with guilt and shame as two words in my vocabulary and life experience. I am choosing to reclaim the joy that I am, and release the fear that keeps me chained to my work, my computer and to a work week that doesn't have days off. Without this I can't be who I want to be in the world, and I certainly can't teach people about self-love, balance, and living in accordance with nature.

What is this incessant need to do? To always be doing, doing, doing? Afraid that life might forget about me if I stop for a few minutes, sit on the couch and have a cup of tea?

The balance of giving and receiving is so crucial to health. I have always been a giver. The shadow side of this is that I have also been a pleaser and have sacrificed my own health, peace, and well-being for others to get or do what they want to. This is not giving. This is self-sabotage disguised in a pretty package with a tag attached saying, "This gift is for you. I hope you like it because I almost killed myself trying to give you everything—my time, energy, money and life force. Love, the Martyr."

My Martyr was really a split personality, flip-flopping back and forth between martyrdom and victimhood. It's time to retire both of those roles and step into true giving, empowerment and self-respect. This means saying no to things or people that may not be in alignment with who I am or what will really serve my highest good. Selfish? Certainly not. I can't truly give until my cup is overflowing with abundance to share. Otherwise, depletion is inevitable.

I write this in the early morning hours, looking out over a glassy lake that reflects a striking snow capped mountain. Here I am. I'm doing it, putting aside all of the excuses that I don't have enough time or money to be here taking two days away from home and work to get a different perspective and reconnect with myself in nature.

This is the change.
This is the self-care.
This is the love I am cultivating.

Chapter 13

Spring Routines

What you may have nurtured in silence over the Winter is now ready to take flight. What you have prayed for, incubated, and built is now open for transformation and freedom. Spring is the season of renewal and simply letting go. The theme for our daily practice is beauty and simplicity. Less is lighter, freer, and inspired. Daily rhythms bring awareness and trust in letting go.

Can you feel the shifts, the opening joyful abandon of each day? Enjoy and observe the changes in your body, mind, and attitude as Spring unfolds and expands your life.

Springtime can trick us into abandoning our daily practice as we feel the need to shed everything and throw out what is no longer needed. Sometimes, we tend to lose ourselves as we crave complete freedom. True liberation comes from implementing our daily rituals and simple practices that free our mind from distractions and impulsive actions that may not be beneficial in the long run. So how do you have freedom and routine at the same time? The answer is to choose and implement the practices and attitudes that will serve and sustain you over time.

Begin simply as always. Shift your practices to a lighter more subtle "Springy" space. Move, laugh, play, explore, experiment, and expand! The Spring daily practices will give you the foundation to leap forward with confidence and the renewed courage of your convictions.

1. Start by waking a little earlier, by about half an hour. If you were waking in Winter at 7 a.m., you can slowly transition into waking at 6:45 a.m., and finally at 6:30 a.m.

    Always allow yourself enough time to do your morning practices without feeling stressed or rushed.

2. Morning cleansing rituals—scrape tongue, brush teeth, and practice oil-pulling.

3. Drink warm water with a squeeze of lemon and an optional 1/2 inch piece of grated ginger. This will clear out Spring congestion from the tissues, assist elimination, and activate digestion.

4. Beautiful Body and Happy Mind Spring Practices:

    - Meditate (even five minutes is a good start).

    - Breathe. Follow your Spring *pranayama* practice.

- Move. Follow your Spring yoga practice or get your body moving in other ways like dancing, bike riding, or brisk walking. Increased activity in Spring helps to move stagnation and congestion, and cleanses the body for the day. Go outside and walk amongst the flowers, inhale the fragrant Spring air. Commune with Nature!

- Self-massage with a blend of warm sesame and sunflower oil, alternating every other day with body scrubs (recipe in Spring self-care section). Take a warm shower while using a natural herbal soap.

- Anoint yourself with aromatic, enlivening, and cleansing essential oils for the Spring. Choose from ginger, cardamom, eucalyptus, rosemary, fennel, sandalwood, lavender, spikenard, basil (see Spring self-care section for applications).

5. Meals: Breakfast, lunch, and dinner taken at the same time each day will facilitate cleansing and encourage a pattern of good digestion. Dry, light meals are best in the Spring with a focus on bitter, pungent, and astringent tastes. Warming herbs and spices cleanse the tissues. Avoid cold foods and oily, heavy foods such as excess dairy, avocados, and/or nuts.

   - Breakfast: Light and nourishing, eaten by 10 a.m.

   - Lunch: Main meal of the day and eaten around midday. Avoid over-eating. Take a short brisk walk after lunch to aid digestion.

   - Dinner: Light, warming, and freshly prepared ideally by 6:30 p.m. Avoid heavy foods in the evening as this can result in congestion and poor, heavy or dull sleep.

   Eat all meals away from your computer, TV, and other electronic distractions.

6. Before bed take some quiet time with at least one hour of distraction-free space. Meditate, journal, pray, chant. Choose an activity that integrates your day and brings a peaceful night sleep. Quality rest rejuvenates and relaxes the body and mind. Aim for bedtime between 10 p.m. and 11 p.m.

   Avoid sleeping during the day as this makes the body feel heavy and congested. Encourage and invite love, romance, and simplicity—after all this is Spring!

Chapter 14

Spring Food Practices

When Spring arrives we are ready to lighten up our diets and our attitudes. We get a feeling of rebirth and recommitting to our health. The idea of a "Spring Cleanse" is in the air and soon we are all cleaning out our pantries, closets, and flushing out our bodies.

Spring harvests provide us with the perfect food for cleansing the liver and clearing congestion in the lungs. As it is rainy, damp, and heavy, Spring offers a natural pharmacopeia of bitter, light greens and detoxifying foods that are low-mucous and low-fat. This diet flushes out the *kapha* that has accumulated in our bodies during the Winter.

Don't you just love Spring? Everything is so fragrant and it feels so good to lighten up. Markets are bursting with flowers, herbs, and sprouts. Walking through the Farmers' Market, find your favourite local farmer who sells vitamin-rich pea shoots and other sprouted greens. Relish munching on them as you walk through the market admiring the flowers, multitude of fresh greens, and other Spring fare.

It is best to avoid heavy, oily, sweet, and sour foods that clog the system while it is trying to melt away toxins. Focusing on foods that will not conflict with the purification and renewal process is the way to go to ensure the channels of the body are kept clear.

What happens to our body and mind in the Spring? After the Winter, the body may have stored up excess fat and mucus, which needs to be moved through and out of the system. *Flush!* In the Spring, the body's wisdom starts to release any stored excess *kapha* or congestion. Everything around us assists in this task. Externally, snow is melting, and internally, things are softening and liquefying getting ready to exit the body. Bye bye!

We can simply observe the foods that are present in the markets and gardens to know what we need to do. The heavy, damp, cool, and liquid qualities of the season are those akin to the earth and water elements. To bring balance we need to eat light, dry, warm, and cleansing foods.

The tastes to focus on in the Spring are bitter, pungent, and astringent.

Nature's fare is abundant in fresh bitter greens such as dandelion, cilantro, parsley, chard, kale, spinach, mustard greens, and arugula to name a few. Lighter grains are best. Use quinoa, millet, amaranth, buckwheat, brown basmati rice, and rye. As everything is popping up all around us, sprouting is a wonderful way to lighten the Winter weight. It is also such a youthful pleasure to watch various sprouting boxes in the kitchen. It makes you feel like a kid connecting to the miracle of new life.

As always, healthy fats are important to include in your diet in every season and in the Spring you can enjoy lighter oils such as flax, canola, sunflower, and mustard oil. The intention for a balanced Spring food practice is light, fresh, and easy.

Tip: Avoid cold, heavy, sweet, and oily foods as they drive toxins deeper into the tissues and create further congestion in the body. Avoid heavy dairy foods such as ice cream, cold milk, yoghurt, and cheese. Spring congestion is aggravated by food and drink that creates overload in the respiratory and digestive system, and literally sticks to the tissues.

Tonic: Bitter tonics and teas are Spring miracles for the mind and body! Enjoy teas consisting of dandelion, nettle, cilantro, fennel, and chamomile. Take a quarter cup of edible aloe vera gel or juice in the morning before your breakfast and munch on sprouts as a snack in the afternoon instead of heavy milky teas and sweets.

Treat: A warm bright, sweet, and spicy juice with a hint of bitter for balance is a delicious afternoon snack. Juice two apples, half a bunch of parsley, one inch fresh ginger, a handful of dandelion or arugula leaves, and half a lemon. Make your own, or find a great juice bar in your neighborhood to make one for you.

Spring Food Guide

Herb and Spice Magic for the Spring

Ajwan	Allspice	Anise	Asafoetida	Basil
Black Pepper	Caraway	Cardamom	Cayenne	Cinnamon
Cloves	Coriander	Cumin	Fennel	Ginger
Garlic	Marjoram	Mustard Seeds	Nutmeg	Orange Peel
Oregano	Paprika	Parsley	Peppermint	Rosemary
Saffron	Sage	Star anise	Tarragon	Thyme
Turmeric				

Spring Legumes

Aduki Beans	Black Beans	Black-Eyed Peas	Chickpeas	Lentils
Lima Beans	Mung Beans	Navy Beans	Pinto Beans	Soybeans
Split Peas	Sprouted beans (all)	Tofu		

Spring Grains

Amaranth	Barley	Buckwheat	Basmati rice (white or brown)	
Corn	Millet	Oats	Quinoa	Rye
Wild Rice				

Spring Fruits

Apples	Apricots	Berries (seasonal)	Dried Fruits	Pears

Spring Veggies

Arugula	Artichoke	Asparagus	Beets	Bell Peppers
Bok Choy	Broccoli	Burdock	Carrots	Cauliflower
Celery	Collards	Daikon	Eggplant	Endive
Fennel	Green Beans	Jicama	Kale	Leeks
Mustard Greens	Okra	Onion	Parsley	Peas
Peppers	Salad Greens: Lettuce, Pea Shoots, Peppercress, Watercress, Chard etc.			
Spinach	Spring Onions	Sprouts (all)	*Squash	*Sweet potato

*In moderation

Spring Dairy

| Ghee | Goats Cheese | Goats Milk | Yoghurt (spiced) |

Spring Fish and Meat

Chicken	Eggs	Fresh Water and Ocean Fish
Lamb (moderation)	Shrimp/Shellfish	Turkey

Spring Nuts Seeds and Condiments

Almonds	Coconut	Hemp Nuts	Pumpkin Seeds
Sesame Seeds	Sunflower Seeds	Spirulina	

Spring Oils

Canola	Flax	Ghee	Mustard	Olive
*Sesame				

*In moderation

Spring Sweeteners

| Honey (raw is best) | Maple Syrup | Molasses | Unrefined cane sugar |

Spring Teas

Burdock Root	Cardamom	Dandelion	Echinacea	Ginger
Lemon	Nettle	*CCF (Classic Ayurvedic tea of cumin, coriander and fennel)		

*To make CCF tea take 1 tsp each of fennel seed, cumin seed, and coriander seed. Add along with 4 cups water to a small pot and bring to boil. When mixture has reached a boil, turn down to simmer for 10-15 minutes. Strain and drink. This tea is cleansing, aids the digestive system and supports the absorption of nutrients in the body while bringing the body into a state of acid/alkaline (pH) balance. A great tea to reset the body after any over-indulgences.

Spring Meal Ideas and Recipes

Breakfast: Toasted oats are wonderful in Spring when everything is so moist and dense. Toast oats lightly in a dry pan until they are slightly browned. Add boiled water at a one-to-one ratio and stir. Allow to sit for five minutes off the heat. Add spices, seeds, nuts, and dried fruits from your Spring Food Guide for a lighter breakfast. Dry, light, and warm foods are best for this damp season.

- Savory breakfasts such as quinoa or millet with sprouts and pungent spices are a good breakfast booster.

- Enjoy poached or boiled eggs with sprouts on rye toast.

- Try a breakfast of berries topped with unsweetened granola and a dollop of cinnamon-spiced yoghurt.

Lunch: This is best as your main meal of the day as digestion is at its prime between noon and 2 p.m.

- Remember to include all six tastes for a balanced and satisfying meal.
- Light dry grains, beans and veggies, or a small portion of animal food makes a good lunch.
- Experiment with a variety of foods from the Spring Food Guide.

Dinner: This can be a lighter meal taken at least three hours before bedtime.

- Enjoy a variety of spices and condiments with your meal to include all six tastes.
- Spring soups, grains, small portions of animal foods, and a rotating variety of veggies is best.
- Simplicity is key for your daily evening meal. Focus on the bitter, pungent, and astringent tastes.
- Eat slowly, enjoy every bite. Offer a prayer of thanks before the meal.

Spring Pasta

Pasta comes in many forms these days. Wheat is too heavy in the Spring, however you can choose from corn, rice, soba, and quinoa noodles found in many natural foods grocery stores. These are lighter and easier to digest at this time of year.

Serves 4

3 cups dry pasta: use quinoa, rice, soba or corn pasta (elbow, spiral, penne, or other fun shapes)
12 cups water to cook pasta
1 tsp olive oil to add to cooking pasta
1 tbsp mustard or olive oil
1 clove chopped garlic
2 cups chopped asparagus pieces
1 cup chopped snap peas
1 tbsp minced spring onions,
1 tbsp minced fresh ginger
1/4 cup finely chopped fennel bulb

Pesto dressing

2 tbsp olive oil
1/2 cup cold water
1 tsp minced tarragon or oregano
1/2 cup chopped fresh basil
2 tbsp sunflower seeds
Pinch of black pepper
1 tsp sea salt
Juice from 1/2 a lemon

1. Boil water to cook pasta, add pasta and 1 tsp olive oil. Be careful not to overcook.

2. When pasta is ready, drain in a colander and give a quick rinse with cold water to wash off the starch.

3. Prepare pesto. In a blender add your tarragon or oregano, basil, sunflower seeds, water, olive oil, lemon juice, black pepper, and salt. Blend until smooth and creamy. Add more water if necessary. Set aside.

4. Heat mustard or olive oil in a pan. Add the chopped garlic, ginger, and fennel and sauté for 2 minutes. Add chopped asparagus, chopped snap peas, and minced spring onions. Sauté together for a few minutes until tender but not overcooked.

5. Add cooked pasta to veggies and sauté together for another 30 seconds melding well.

6. Turn heat off and add pesto. Mix together well and enjoy!

7. This easy and delicious pasta idea can include a variety of other Spring veggies and herbs for a quick and easy meal. Also consider adding any other Spring protein such as fish or beans or tofu to the sauté if you desire a fuller meal.

Everybody's Spring *Kichari*

To sprout or not to sprout? The following is a recipe for a lovely Spring *kichari* which can be enlivened even more if you sprout the whole mung beans ahead of time. Try it both ways and decide for yourself!

Serves 4

4 tbsp ghee
1 tsp cumin seeds
1 tsp coriander seeds

1 tsp fennel seeds
Half a medium onion finely diced
1 inch fresh peeled ginger, finely diced
1/4 tsp asafoetida (optional—a good addition though as this reduces the gaseous nature of beans)
1 cup split mung dal (sprouted whole mung beans as an option for a lighter *kichari*)*
3/4 cup white basmati rice
1/2 bunch spinach (alternatively, 1-2 cups of other greens or veggies such as asparagus, zucchini, daikon or a combination)
1 1/2 tsp sea salt/rock salt
6 cups water (may add more water for a more watery *kichari*, or less for a drier stew)

1. Soak split mung beans and rice together in cold water overnight.

2. In a heavy-bottomed pan, heat the ghee on medium and add the onions and ginger to sauté until tender.

3. Add the cumin, fennel and coriander seeds and sauté for 2 more minutes.

4. Add the asafoetida and stir in.

5. Drain the split mung beans and rice until the rinse water is clear, and add to the mixture.

6. Sauté for a few more minutes and add the water, cover, and bring to a boil.

7. Once boiling, stir, lower heat, and simmer with the lid on until tender (about 20 minutes).

8. While the *kichari* is cooking, wash and chop the spinach/greens.

9. Add the greens to the top of the mixture and replace the cover. Allow to steam on top for 1-2 minutes if using spinach, and 3-5 minutes for other veggies.

10. Stir in, add salt, and mix in.

11. Garnish with a squeeze of lime, fresh cilantro or parsley, a small dollop more of ghee, and toasted sesame seeds. You can also sprinkle some desiccated coconut on top.

*If sprouting mung beans: use whole mung beans and rinse in cold water until water is clear. Cover beans with cold water until all beans are well immersed. Soak overnight for at least 8-12 hours. Discard soaking water and rinse well with cold water. Place in colander out of direct sunlight and leave to drain for 8 more hours. You will notice tiny sprouts popping up.

You can use them to cook into *kichari* at this stage or rinse and drain for another 8 hours for longer sprouts.

Spring Cleansing Veggie Mineral Broth

A must-have! This savory broth is not only cleansing, but also nourishing, and full of easy-to-digest vitamins and minerals. Get into the habit every time you cook to save your veggie peelings, seeds, and skins. Whether you are peeling root veggies, removing kale or collard leaves from the stalks, scraping carrot skins, trimming the edges off squashes, peeling onions—have a plastic bag ready and save the cuttings. Not for the compost bin—oh no! You want to save these in your fridge (for up to a week) or in your freezer if longer, to make a satisfying broth. This will become your best-friend-in-a-flask, we promise!

How to make your broth:

- In a large pot add 12-16 cups of water plus all the veggie peelings, skins, seeds, etc.
- Bring all to a boil. You can add additional chunky-cut veggies for a richer broth.
- Simmer on low with lid partially on for 45 minutes. Strain. Add salt as needed.

Some veggies you may want to add to your broth in addition to the peelings: carrots, beets, celery, parsley, dandelion, cilantro, ginger, and arugula. You can also add dulce, kelp or other sea vegetables as they are rich in iron as well as Vitamin C, which increases the bioavailability of iron in the body.

Sip your broth whenever feeling in need of a pick-me-up. Just pour yourself a cup and exhale while visualizing your tissues being revitalized and your body being flushed of toxins.

Spring Beddy-bye Tonic for a Good Sleep

To be enjoyed a half an hour before bed.

Brew a cup of a bitter/pungent herbal tea such as dandelion, burdock root, cardamom, or ginger. There are many varieties of herbal teas available to choose from. Add a touch of honey for sweetness. Honey is a miracle food for Springtime as it strips away toxins from the tissues and removes phlegm from the lungs.

This tea will clear the mind and assist in clearing out any congestion in the system to allow for a restful nights sleep.

Chapter 15

Spring Self-Care

After Winter, we emerge from the still dark days and embrace all that this season of promise has to offer. Beauty is everywhere, and as the excesses and toxins are released, so we make room for Nature's gift of renewal.

G

I love this inspired Navajo prayer that I first learned at a rainbow gathering in Oregon many years ago while attending a ceremony with First Nation elders. I find it brings awareness and a connection to something greater. Say it out loud in a forest, by the ocean, in a meadow of flowers, in your garden, in your sacred home space. Awaken yourself to the glory of Spring, and appreciate your own unique beauty.

May it be beautiful before me.

May it be beautiful below me.

May it be beautiful behind me.

May it be beautiful above me.

May it be beautiful all around me.

I am restored in beauty.

I am restored in beauty.

I am restored in beauty.

I am restored in beauty.

With Spring being the kapha *time of year, this season in particular evokes the sense of taste and smell. My morning walk is perfumed with lilacs, tea roses, and honeysuckle. As I step forward and bury my nose in a halo of aromatic wonder, I can feel the perfume flow through my nasal passages, fill my lungs, and touch every part of my insides with its fragrant beauty.*

> *I visualize this perfume purifying and blessing every tissue, cell, and organ inside my body and surrounding me with a radiant haze. This simple aromatic visualization practice always brings me joy and fills me with the beauty of the flower itself.*

Try this aromatic breathing ritual! You will feel confident exuding this floral scent wherever you go. Others will notice.

These simple self-care practices keep you in the flow of this gorgeous season and can assist in moving out the stuff you no longer need in your life. This gives you the space to pay attention to the more sustainable possessions such as radiant health, inner beauty, and grace.

Choose the ones that speak to you. Make the transition from your Winter practices, and stock your apothecary with the Spring potions and elixirs that will be your companions for renewal and glowing health until Summer comes.

Spring Flowers Face Cleanse

Put your best face forward. Cleansing the channels of the body also includes purifying the skin, the body's largest organ of elimination. At this time of year, our face is ready for some exfoliation and refreshment. Ground nuts, seeds, and flowers are the ideal tools for this cleansing ritual and green tea is an additional astringent tonic.

Make enough to have a week or two supply of this regenerating cleanser to keep skin supple, soft, and dewy. Use it in the morning to gently cleanse your skin.

Dry ingredients

1 cup white basmati rice, ground into a powder in an electric grinder (or mortar and pestle, should you be so inspired)
1/4 cup dried ground rose petals or lavender petals, finely ground
1 tsp dried green tea (optional), finely crushed leaves or powder
(Blend together and store in an airtight glass jar in a cool dry place or in the refrigerator)

Wet ingredients

1/4 tsp apricot kernel oil
1/4 tsp plain fresh organic yoghurt (Keep separate, and measure and add to dry mix to make into a paste for each cleansing application)

For your daily morning face cleansing ritual:

1. Take a tbsp of the dry mixture and add to apricot kernel oil and fresh yoghurt (add water if needed to make into a smooth consistency).

2. Mix into a paste and with upward sweeping and circular strokes massage over entire neck and face. Add more liquid if necessary to get a smoother application.

3. Without scrubbing, gently massage face all over with this aromatic, nutrient-rich, cleansing feast.

4. Wash off with warm water and gently pat skin dry with a clean towel.

Springtime Moisturizer

Make enough for a week or two supply of this light moisturizer.
Use in the morning to moisturize, revitalize, and brighten your skin for the day.

1 cup unrefined apricot oil
12 drops bergamot essential oil (EO)
6 drops clary sage EO
6 drops lavender EO
1 small bottle of orange blossom water or regular witch hazel toner to have on hand. (Do not mix into oil blend—keep separate)

Mix the apricot oil and the essential oils together well and store in an airtight glass bottle.

Each morning after cleansing, take 1/4 tsp of the oil blend and mix with 1 tsp witch hazel toner. Massage into face.

Spring Shower Lover

Make enough for a week or two supply of this skin-detoxifying, joy-enhancing, aromatic body scrub to play with in the shower. The scrub is rich in purifying mineral salts, astringent herbs, and oils to beautify your skin.

4 cups fine Himalayan sea salt
1/2 cup almond oil
1/2 cup sunflower oil
6 drops bergamot EO
6 drops basil EO
6 drops ginger EO
6 drops rosemary EO
1/4 cup of ground rose petals (optional)

Stir salts, oils, rose petals and essential oils to richly and lavishly coat the salt grains. Add to a glass jar with a seal and sit near bathtub so you can grab the mix whenever your skin needs a shower lover.

Tip: Stand in shower. Wet skin. Turn off water or step away from the water flow. Grab a handful of the oily salt scrub and lightly rub over body. Turn water back on and rinse. The body will have a thin coating of the oil and feel soft and supple all day. Treat yourself to this at least once a week in the mornings!

Spring-in-Your-Step Elixir

This drink is cleansing, detoxing, and energizing—a happy triad of health for Spring. This elixir has a bitter component for cleansing, and also a slightly sweet and pungent taste for stimulating digestion and increasing circulation. An amazing afternoon boost for your liver.

Juice:

1 bunch parsley
1 inch fresh ginger
1 beet
2 stalks celery
1 lemon
A pinch of cayenne pepper

A juicer is a wonderful kitchen helper. If you don't have a juicer locate a juice bar that makes fresh organic juices. Avoid sweetened, store-bought juices.

Pucker up, because as bitter as this tonic may be, you will be feeling so great that you are going to want to celebrate with a kiss!

Scents of Spring: Aromatherapy

Every season brings an opportunity to make friends with the healing plant essences!

In the Spring, we use essential oils to balance the wet, cool, and heavy qualities of the season that can affect our body and make us feel sluggish, depressed, and lethargic. Aromatherapy soothes the mind and brings equilibrium to the emotions and can miraculously transform your relationship to everything within and around you. It is a subtle but effective way to boost your self-esteem and detox your system in cooperation with the natural rhythms of the season.

Slowly build your aromatherapy apothecary for each season and you will always have a remedy on hand. The oils are versatile and can be blended in a multitude of ways.

Your nose knows!

Suggested Essential Oil List for Spring
(Inspiring, vitalizing, decongesting, astringent, pungent, detoxifying)

Stock your bathroom apothecary with at least three or four of these fragrant friends:

ginger, cardamom, eucalyptus, rosemary, fennel, black pepper, clary sage, bergamot, oregano, sweet orange, sage, juniper, cinnamon, lavender, rose, basil, spikenard, sandalwood, lemongrass, lemon.

How to apply aromatherapy to your daily Spring practice:

Make a pure essential oil blend using two or three of the different oils listed. Store in a dark, airtight glass bottle. You can also keep four or five different essential oils in your bathroom cabinet and blend as needed or use individually as preferred.

1. Massage oil: By adding an essential oil blend to a carrier oil, you can have a customized massage blend on hand to use as needed. Two lovely massage carrier oils for the Spring are sunflower or almond oil or an equal mix of the two. A ratio of approximately 48-90 drops (total) of pure essential oil to 4 oz carrier oil is the standard range depending on how potent you want your blend. Keep your blend simple when starting out by using only three or four essential oils. Play and experiment as you discover the best scents for you.

2. Bath oil: The best way to use essential oils in the bath is to mix them with salts or an emulsifier such as milk (think Cleopatra) or your carrier oil. You can also add your custom massage blend directly into the bath. Two to three tablespoons of your blend would make for a luxurious bath allowing the oils to be absorbed deeply into the skin.

   A good ratio is 10-20 drops essential oil, mixed with 1/2 cup of salt or emulsifier.

Aromatic baths in the Spring are excellent for the respiratory system, as well as for relieving stress and detoxifying the system.

3. Direct Palm Inhalation: Apply 1-2 drops of essential oil directly to the palms, rub together gently and inhale deeply. This is an excellent method to use for a quick and easy exposure to the benefits of the essential oils.

4. Facial steam: Put 1-3 drops total of essential oils in a bowl of steaming hot water, cover head with a towel, and steam face. Excellent for opening sinuses and clearing congestion. Eucalyptus, basil, and rosemary are particularly good at this time of year.

G & M's Spring Journals

G

May 25th

Blank.

Sometimes I so badly want to express my thoughts, feelings, and words, and I come up with nothing. An explosion may be going on inside and it feels trapped, stuck, pushing against the walls of my cells, knocking to come out, and nothing. Creativity seems to be blocked and I come to a standstill. This is something that cannot be forced, extruded, pulled or pushed. When this happens I remind myself what to do. I close my eyes, breathe and just make space. It can take minutes, or an hour, or a week, but I allow a softening and I just stop the fight inside.

I think of the wise and lovable Yoda from Star Wars and his sage advice, "Do or do not, there is no try."

So I do not.

When these times come I sit in a place of non-judgment, understanding that the wisdom of "there is no try" really means not to go into anything with half hearted intent. Just do it! Or do not.

It is so uncomfortable for a driven, ambitious, over-achieving, pitta *perfectionist to "do not."*

When my resources are drained, my energy is low, and my heart is not in it, I remind myself to not try and push the river. When I fight against the flow of what my body and mind need I come up with something that is not authentic.

So I turn my attention elsewhere to rejuvenate, enliven, energize, and get back in the creative flow.

M

May 5th

Nothing is guaranteed.

Of course, I've known this in theory and even talked about it with great clarity in my yoga classes, but I never used to think this really applied to me. It is liberating and confining for me to live in the abyss so conveniently cloaked in the veil of regularity. The sun comes up everyday; we all go about our business and the sun sets . . . I've become attached to believing that things are permanent (at least temporarily permanent), that my parents, friends and sun will always be here.

As I walked down to the ocean today, I became very present to everything around me. I smelled a rose growing between the thorny blackberry bushes. I felt the rocks with my fingertips. I really saw, with all of my senses, the ever-changing water of the ocean as she lapped her sweet power upon the sand. I saw a half-eaten seal and again I was brought back to the impermanence of everything.

I smiled at people as I walked up the hill. I made eye contact with strangers. I felt the crisp Spring air on my checks and I whispered softly to myself, "Thank you."

I am so grateful for this day.

Chapter 16

Spring Yoga, *Pranayama*, and Meditation

Spring Yoga Practice: Just Do It!

Springtime yoga is all about getting up and moving. Move it. Shake it. Get your blood flowing. Thaw out from the heaviness and introspection of Winter, and blossom into the radiant expression of magnificence that you are.

Reduce excess *kapha* through your daily yoga practice by flowing through the postures. Increase the dynamic, heating, and light qualities to energize, detoxify, and balance your body and mind.

> **Spring Flow Tips**
>
> ~ Be consistent.
> ~ Generate routine by practicing at the same time everyday.
> ~ Ideal time to practice: mornings, between sunrise and 10 a.m.
> ~ Anytime is better than not at all.
> ~ Manage your energy with calm and steady breathing in and out through your nose, or use *ujjayi* breath throughout your practice.
> ~ Tap into your inner child: be playful, enthusiastic, and light-hearted.

Yoga Time

As mentioned, the ideal time to do your yoga practice in the Spring is in the early morning. You want to generate a light sweat to assist in the detoxification of the body through the skin. Move more vigorously to enliven and energize yourself. Put on some uplifting music if that helps you to wake up and move!

On those days that you would rather push the snooze button one more time, give yourself an Ayurvedic kick in the pants, connect to your fire centre, and empower yourself with the gift of yoga.

You know you will be glad that you did!

For the Spring, focus on the ancient practice of *surya namaskara*, the sun salutation. Do this repeatedly. Do this flow like your life depends on it. Do it with enthusiasm and commitment. Do this now.

Surya namaskara is so well-rounded, it is an entire practice within itself. It benefits your digestion, circulation, immunity, respiration, lymph flow, and detoxification.

Without the Sun, life could not exist on this planet. *Surya* means "sun" and *namaskara* is, "to pay homage to." This practice honours life, the giver of life, and the rising spiritual sun (consciousness) within.

Surya namaskara is a dance, a prayer, and a humble offering acknowledging the sustainer. Ideally, face East, the direction of the rising sun when doing your practice.

Surya Namaskara: Sun Salutation

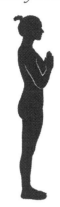
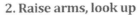

1. Standing pose
Stand with your feet together and hands in *pranam mudra* (prayer mudra) with palms together in front of the heart. Inhale, exhale.

2. Raise arms, look up
Inhale as you raise your arms out to the sides and overhead. Look up while keeping the back of your neck elongated.

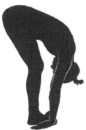

3. Forward fold
Exhale as you bend from the hips, tilting the pelvis forward. Bring the chest parallel to the thighs—bend your knees if you feel tightness in your hamstrings or back.

4. Lunge
Inhale, step your right leg back, lower your right knee onto the floor and place your fingertips beside your front heel, or place your hands on your thigh. Lift your chest and keep your spine long.

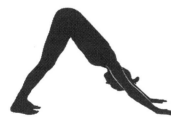

5. Down dog
Exhale, step your right foot back so that both of your hands are pressing into the floor. Feet are parallel, hip distance apart, and your sitting bones are pointing up towards the sky. Keep your head in line with your spine. Take one inhalation here.

6. Eight-Point Salute
Exhale, lower your knees, chest, and chin to the floor all at once (for a simpler version lower your knees to the ground first), keeping your buttocks high in the sky.

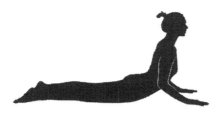

7. Cobra
Inhale, slide your chest along the ground past your hands and then lift your chest up off of the floor to a comfortable degree.

8. Down dog
Exhale, shift the weight of your body (especially the pelvis) back and up until both of your hands are pressing into the floor, feet are parallel and hip distance apart. Your sitting bones are pointing up towards the sky. Keep your head in line with your spine.

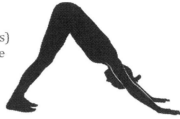

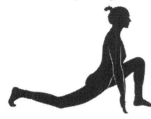

9. Lunge
Inhale, keep your pelvis lifted up high to make room to step your left foot forward in between your hands. Return to your lunge position with your fingertips beside your front heel or place your hands on your thighs. Lift your chest and keep your spine long.

10. Forward fold
Exhale, step your back foot forward to meet your front foot, returning to your forward fold, bending at the hips, belly button touching the thighs (again, bend your knees if you feel tightness in your hamstrings or back).

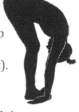

11. Raise arms, look up
Inhale as you lift your torso, raise your arms out to the sides and then overhead. Look up while keeping the back of your neck elongated.

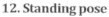

12. Standing pose
Exhale, bring your palms back together in *pranam mudra*. Inhale. Repeat on the second side. The only difference is in the lunge. On the second side, take your left leg back and then for the second lunge in the sequence step your right foot forward (so that your left leg remains back).

Now you have completed one full round.

Start by doing nine rounds, and work your way up to 27 rounds every morning. Have fun! Tap into the life-giving energy of *Surya*.

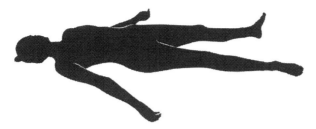

13. Icing on the Cake (*Savasana*—Corpse Pose)
(2-4 min.)
Sorry to be the bearer of this news, however if you have more *kapha* in your constitution, you, my friend, must only take a couple of deep restful minutes so that you don't slip back into never-never-land (for *kapha* types love to sleep!)

Lay down on your back with your head and spine straight, legs apart, letting the feet flop out to the sides. Arms are away from the sides of the body slightly and the palms face upward.

Close your eyes.

Let your entire body relax. Begin at your toes and relax your feet. Move your awareness up through the body all the way to the head, consciously letting go of any stress or tension along the way. Your breath should be completely natural. Surrender into the stillness and silence of this posture.

Once you have completed the practice, start to wiggle your fingers and toes. Stretch your body in any way that feels great. Roll to one side, and use your hands to push yourself to an upright position.

Honour Yourself

Take a moment to observe how you are feeling physically, mentally, emotionally, and energetically after your yoga practice.

Thank yourself for doing the practice (gratitude expands more of what we want in our life).

Honour your strengths and weaknesses of mind and body. Self-acceptance goes a long way.

Practice Tips

- If this is a new practice to you, learn it in stages. For example, take the first five steps of the sequence and get to know them really well before gradually adding more and more of the postures. Before you know it you will have the entire flow of *surya namaskara* and can use it as a warm up anytime, anywhere.

- As *surya namaskara* is a dynamic, invigorating practice, doing this in the evening before bed may be too stimulating.

Spring *Pranayama*: Shine that skull! What?

Breath is life.

In the Spring, we thaw out and prepare for a rebirth of sorts. The first action a baby takes in this world is of inhalation. As infants, we draw in a new life with breath: We bring in the *prana*, the essential energetic expression of existence. We are propelled forward into being. The energy of Spring invites us to let go in order to rebirth, recreate, and renew.

Pranayama practices have a powerful psycho-biological effect, enhancing both the quality of a cellular structure and releasing toxins on a mental level, thus restructuring our body and mind to be more aligned with incredible vitality and increased positivity.

Kapalbhati is translated as the "skull shining breath." This *pranayama* practice has the medicinal qualities of creating heat and thus detoxifying the organs by flushing fresh oxygen into our system. In the Springtime, we can assist our bodies to detoxify from the accumulation of heaviness after a long Winter of eating richer foods and spending more time indoors.

This breathing technique helps to remove impurities both mentally and physically, particularly in the lungs. It is very good if you have asthma, bronchitis, or mucous congestion. *Kapalbhati* strengthens the nervous system, reduces stress, fortifies immunity, increases mental clarity, and energizes the whole system. If you are feeling heavy, sluggish, depressed, or tired, kick up a round of *kapalbhati* instead of reaching for that cup of coffee.

In yogic terms this *pranayama* cleanses both *ida* and *pingala nadis* (the energy channels relating to the two hemispheres of the brain) and clears out toxic *ama* in the mind and body. It is a heating and stimulating practice so it is not one to practice before bedtime or if you are already overheated. Also, if you have heart disease, high blood pressure, ulcer, stroke, hernia, or epilepsy be sure to get the green light from your doctor before beginning practice.

The How-To of *Kapalbhati* Breathing

1. Sit in a comfortable position in a chair, with your back against the wall, or cross-legged—wherever you can have an elongated spine.

2. Establish a slow, calm, and steady breathing pattern in and out of your nostrils.

3. Take a deep breath in. Halfway through your exhalation begin to forcefully exhale and simultaneously contract the abdominal muscles (imagine you're blowing out a candle with your nose).

4. Allow your inhalation to be passive and effortless, and the belly will naturally expand.

5. Continue for 10 more breaths.

6. Pause. Take a natural breath before commencing 10 more.

Practice Tips

- The exhalation is rhythmic, sharp, and short.

- If you feel light-headed at any time, take a break.

- Once you are familiar and comfortable with the practice you can increase the number of rounds that you do, up to 20 rounds of 10 exhalations.

Meditation for Spring: Walking Towards Enlightenment

M

My Grandmother lived to the ripe age of 103. One day I asked her, "Grandma, what is your secret to living such a long and healthy life?" She claimed there was no secret, not one that she thought of as anything out of the ordinary, that is.

Nevertheless, the way she consistently lived her life was in balance. The kind of balance that is so natural and organic that it is effortless.

My Grandmother had no interest in yoga, meditation, or high falutin philosophy, yet she lived the teachings through her being. She ate a balanced diet, neither indulging nor depriving herself. She laughed daily, always looked on the bright side (after living through two World Wars), and she walked each and every day!

That is it. The secrets to living a long, healthy, and happy life are right there, folks. Seriously, if we could do these four things daily, we would have a healthy society: eat in moderation; laugh; think positively; and walk everyday.

Walking is one of the most underrated sports around. It is not at all sexy, you do not need any fancy equipment to show off, and you don't need any particular unique skills. Taking this practice to the next level, you become an enlightened walker, where walking becomes a form of meditation. When you bring full presence to this pedestrian movement, it becomes glorious and illuminating.

We know you might be thinking, "Yeah, yeah, I know how to walk, let me just skip to the next page and get on with things." This book offers you the challenge to do this meditation and notice how different your experience of walking becomes. Give yourself some time, not when you're rushing off to get groceries or walking your kids to school.

The How-To of the Walking Meditation

1. Start by standing still and taking a few deep breaths to ground and centre yourself.

2. When you feel ready, take a slow inhalation and pick up your right foot.

3. Exhale, as you slowly place the heel down on the ground, then the mid portion of your foot, and finally the ball and toes.

4. Feel the transfer of weight through your foot as your body prepares to pick the left foot off of the ground.

5. Repeat (you get the idea).

Meditation Tips

- Begin practicing this meditation by moving as slowly as you can without falling asleep.

- Stay connected to the breath the entire time.

- Feel every nuance of movement, sensation, and pulsation throughout the body as you move through space.

- Bring a sense of aliveness, of awakened embodiment to this meditation.

Chapter 17

Spring Ceremony and Ritual

G

Springtime is full of delightful and significant ritual and symbolism. Being the season of renewal and rebirth, this is a powerful opportunity to recognize this energy and bring it into being.

I recently celebrated a Passover dinner with friends and I was reminded of why we do this every year. We went around the table, each saying what we considered our ultimate freedom, and we realized how blessed we were to even engage in this conversation.

There are so many symbolic rituals to mark the passage of Spring. Passover which, aligns with Easter and other Spring holidays (either religiously or culturally) is a time of letting go of the old and bringing in the new. Easter can be followed back to the ancient pagan goddess Eostre, who represents the Springtime, the rising sun, fertility, and new life. Eggs play a big part in many of these rituals, as a palpable symbol of fertility and rebirth. Beginning again.

We acknowledge where we have been, and move forward to where we intend to go.

There are powerful rituals where we become aware of the idea of freedom and the basic human right of making choices for our own lives. There are still too many cultures where women have no freedom, and so we acknowledge this ongoing struggle and give gratitude for our own freedom. We must rid ourselves of things that no longer fit so we can be present without being bogged down. There are many rituals that empower us to do so. Above all, when observing and integrating all the rituals of Spring, we are reminded of the importance of personal renewal.

In the Hindu culture, *Holi* is celebrated to mark the beginning of the Spring and acknowledge new life and energy. If you have ever experienced *Holi*, you will know what it is to experience mischief and wild abandon. All over the streets of India, Pakistan, Bangladesh, Laos, and Nepal, coloured powders are flung around at anyone and everyone, and coloured water squirted and sprayed from water guns.

Holi is a festival welcoming the season of renewal, based on intricate religious stories where the moral is that good always wins over evil. The ritual is about love and welcoming a chance for new beginnings.

Holi is also a festival of humility, equality, and joy. No one out on the streets is spared, and this makes it a great equalizer. It is a celebration of great humour and community.

In Ayurveda, we get the opportunity to "begin again" every Spring as the cells renew themselves after a Spring cleanse, naturally facilitated by our bodies during this season. As Ayurveda sees it, the Spring Equinox is the perfect time for *Pancha Karma* or detoxing.

Clear out the old and bring renewal to everything in your life.

All of these Spring rituals are prescribed for beginning anew in a fun and engaging way:

- To awaken a creative outlook on our life.
- To birth new ideas and ways of being.
- To acknowledge our freedoms and have gratitude for our renewal.
- To jump, sing, flirt, create, invent, inspire, and be present.
- To let go of everything if necessary with faith.

We will be replenished no matter what.

Spring Ceremony Themes: Flowers, Colours, and Egg Mandalas

Create your Spring sacred space: flowers, bright joyful objects, poetry that inspires you, candles. Remove all of the Winter objects from your altar and place a new cloth and other meaningful items or just keep it very simple. Your altar, your choice.

Spring rituals inspire us to set ourselves free and awake from the Winter dream renewed. Inspired by the symbolism of eggs to mark the birth of Spring, create an egg mandala which you can adorn with flowers, patterns, symbols in any way you feel drawn to. Use colour, collage, paint, words, wool, fabric, whatever inspires YOU.

The mandala placed within the egg symbol offers insight and sparks the imagination to birth your dreams. You can create as many egg mandalas as you have ideas that you wish to bring forth into the world. Place them on your altar or on the wall in your sacred space. Adorn your altar with flowers. The floral fragrance and beauty will remind you to connect this egg ritual with everything this new season has to offer on your journey!

Feel free to use this egg mandala template for your guide to copy and paste, or create your own!

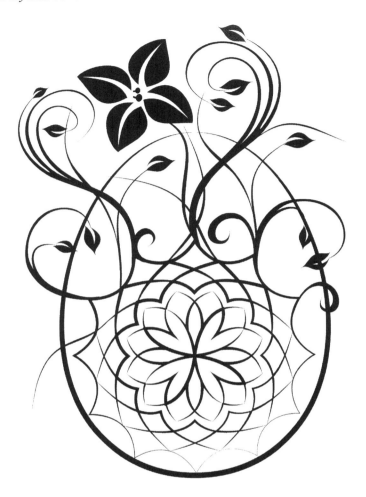

As a sacred environment that is set up and energized with your intentions, your altar acts as the witness, holding the space for your ceremonies and rituals. Once you have set up your personal space for ritual you may find that small miracles begin to happen.

Awakenings may spark new ideas, feelings of joy and motivation.

If you have not already set up your altar space, now is a good time to do so.

Chapter 18

15-Day Sensational Spring Cleanse

Why a Spring Cleanse?

The transition of each season brings a vulnerability to the immune system. It is an opportunity to pause, reset your digestion, your consciousness, and attune yourself to the rhythms of the upcoming season.

Spring being the *kapha* season, we focus on a cleansing practice that pacifies the earth and water elements. As the season is wet, heavy, and dull, the Spring cleanse helps to clear out the excess congestion and mucous that has accumulated throughout the Winter.

A simple mono-diet of *kichari* benefits proper digestion, assimilation, and elimination to regain equilibrium of metabolic function, cleanse the liver and the channels of the body.

This classic Ayurvedic cleansing food is also nourishing, satisfying, and simple. It is a complete protein combination of mung beans and rice. With a little twist for the Spring, sprouted mung beans are lighter, have more nutrients and are aligned with the blossoming of the season. The spices aid in stoking the *agni* (digestive fire), and the ghee assists to dislodge *ama* out and away from the tissues to the digestive tract, where they can be eliminated. Light spring greens complete this perfect detox dish providing fiber, colour, and texture to the experience.

During the season of rebirth, this simple cleanse clears out unwanted gunk and prepares you for a new cycle of possibility and astounding health.

Enjoy the Benefits:

- Improved digestion
- Clear skin
- More energy
- Better sleep
- Healthy weight
- Mental clarity
- Improved focus and memory
- Improved immunity
- Reduce excess mucous
- Increased levels of joy

Shopping List for Everything You Need:

- Basmati rice (the white variety is easiest to digest)
- Mung beans (whole or split)
- Spices: cumin, coriander, fennel, asafoetida and other Spring spices from your Spring Food Guide
- Ghee
- Veggies: spinach, chard, arugula, dandelion greens, and greens of your choice from the Spring Food Guide
- Salt: rock salt or sea salt
- *Triphala*
- Herbal teas: ginger, cardamom, dandelion, burdock and other choices from the Spring Food Guide
- Sunflower oil for self massage

Your Spring Cleanse Calendar

Each Day:

- Scrape your tongue.
- Daily self massage with sunflower oil.
- Incorporate the Spring yoga practice into your day.
- Follow the Spring *pranayama* and meditation practices.
- Consume mineral broths and herbal teas throughout the day (recipe found in the Spring food section).
- Take some quiet time to yourself everyday.
- Take *triphala*, an Ayurvedic herbal formula to assist in gently cleansing and rejuvenating the body.

Days 1-5

Cleanse prep: The first five days prepare you by eliminating trigger foods and foods that are acidic, clogging, and heavy, thus initiating the process of shifting your body to a more alkaline state. During these first five days introduce mineral broth and herbal teas (See Spring Food Guide).

Day 1: Eliminate dairy, (except ghee) alcohol, and sodas.
    Begin taking *triphala*: 1/2 tsp in 1/2 cup warm water at night before bed.

Day 2: Eliminate sugar and animal products.

Day 3: Eliminate coffee, caffeine, and chocolate.

Day 4: Eliminate all processed foods.

Day 5: Eliminate fruit juices, dried fruit, fresh fruit, and nuts.

You are free to choose what foods you eat with the above considerations. For inspiration refer to the Spring Food Guide for the ideal food choices at this time of year.

Days 6-10

You start to shift the body consciousness around eating and your relationship to food by introducing the mono-diet of *kichari*. See *kichari* recipe in Spring Recipe section. Keep smiling.

Day 6: *Kichari* all meals/when hungry. To keep it interesting add condiments. Shredded coconut, cilantro, sprouts (alfalfa, pea tips, sunflower sprouts).

Day 7: *Kichari* all meals/when hungry. Wow Day 7—Rock your cleanse!

Day 8: *Kichari* all meals/when hungry. Get creative with seasonal greens (arugula, dandelion, chard, mustard).

Day 9: *Kichari* all meals/when hungry. You're doing amazing, keep going!

Day 10: *Kichari* all meals/when hungry. Last day of *kichari*!

Days 11-15

Coming out of the cleanse is as important as the cleanse itself.

Reintroduce other healthful foods, but still avoid sugar, caffeine, alcohol, processed foods, chocolate, and dairy.

Chew your food well.

Avoid over-eating.

Days 11-14: Reintroduce a variety of grains (quinoa, barley, brown rice), healthy proteins (nuts, legumes, eggs), fruits (eaten separately from other foods) and vegetables.

Day 15: Final Day. Congrats you did it!

How are you feeling now? Begin to bring more variety into your diet, keeping in mind your daily food practices for the Spring season.

Continue taking *triphala* up to three months if you suffer from indigestion, gas, bloating, or constipation.

Daily Cleanse Check-in

Day	How do you feel today? Physically, mentally, emotionally?	What is your energy level like today? (from 1, lowest, to 10, highest)	What challenges are you currently experiencing?
1			
2			
3			
4			
5			
6			
7			
8			
9			
10			
11			
12			
13			
14			
15			

Part 4

Summer Time

Chapter 19

The Exuberance of Summer

"We don't cease to play because we grow old. We grow old because we cease to play."

~ George Bernard Shaw

M

I absolutely love the Summer!

Growing up I was allowed to play outside with the neighbourhood kids until it got dark. The long Summer evenings seemed to last for years, an eternal game of Kick the Can was bliss for me. Staying up late felt like freedom. Drive-in movie theatres, swimming in the lake, fishing, basking in the sun, summer holidays, camping, barbecues, hanging out with friends—as a kid, Summer was the respite from the hard work the rest of the year (or at least what felt hard when I was eight years old).

There is a certain smell in the air at this time of year and everyone seems to be infused with a lightness that is palpable. Work takes a back seat, and playing is accepted. Down at the beach, kids build sandcastles, teenagers meet to attract a Summer romance, and adults become kids again.

This past year I got a cruiser, a modern take on a sexy 60's surf-culture bicycle. My sparkly, mint green bike with chrome handlebars and big wide seat couldn't make me happier. I never thought that I would consider a bicycle beautiful, keep one in my living room, or shine it everyday . . . but every time I get on my bike, I have an enormous silly grin on my face, and I feel like I'm 10 again.

Perhaps it's not all about the bike but how the cruiser connects me to the part of myself that loves to play, have fun and thinks that life can be easy and joyful; the little girl who still believes that anything is possible . . .

Summer is the time when the sun is highest in the sky and at its brightest. It is no surprise that this coincides with the *pitta* (fire) time of year. *Pitta* is the one *dosha* that has inherent heat. Other qualities which can be used to describe *pitta* types are: light, penetrating, luminous, spreading, oily, inflamed, and mobile. Sometimes *pitta* out of control can be too hot to handle: that bull-headed boss, jealous boyfriend, or inner burning desire to do everything *now!*

For *pitta*, excess heat can burn the midnight oil at both ends, burn others out, or leave a smattering of char-grilled friends and family in the wake of an overzealous control freak. However, in balance, *pitta* is an inspiring leader, holds great wisdom, can light up a room with charismatic clarity, and move mountains with their strong conviction and beliefs.

Pitta literally needs to cool it and chill out on every level and in every way. Take a deep breath, relax, and trust that you don't need to control everything and everyone, and try to have a little bit of fun at the end of the 80-hour work week, okay? That goes for all of us at this time of year.

Summer is the perfect time to remember what is really important in life.

Is it accomplishments . . . or relationships?

Achievement . . . or love?

Ambition . . . or deep connection?

You decide.

When you find yourself in a self-righteous hot-headed *pitta* moment, get on your bike and just ride . . . ride . . . ride.

8 Summer Journal Questions

1. What does the Summer season represent to you?
2. What qualities are invoked within you during the Summer?
3. What you love about the Summer time is . . .
4. What three things can you do for yourself this Summer to stay balanced physically, mentally, and emotionally?
5. Where would you like to direct your energy this season?
6. How can you make this happen?
7. What aspect of yourself is no longer serving you that you are ready to evolve out of?
8. What aspect of yourself would you like to expand?

G & M's Summer Journals

G

June 1st

This morning I woke up on my birthday thinking about some very important people in my life who were taken away at a very young age, way before their time. I got to think what the phrase, "before your time," means because I also believe that when it's your time, it's your time.

One of my closest friends from South Africa was killed in a car accident at the age of 26. Laura was a few years older than me and a powerful role model and mentor for me in my early twenties. She was a shining star. Laura had become increasingly addicted to the calming effects of marijuana. She had smoked some that day, and had gotten into her car thinking that she was in control. It took me years to try and understand why she had become dependent on this powerful herb to make her feel good when she seemed so happy and her life seemed so amazing, successful, and fulfilled. Everything looked perfect from the outside.

I understand now that has nothing to do with it.

Ellen Msimanga, my beloved nanny for 19 years, died of a heart attack at the young age of 48. Ellen's life was filled with joy and faith and also tragic loss. Her son, Mandla, was stabbed to death for the equivalent of five dollars in one of the townships in Johannesburg when he was only 16 years old. Ellen endured the pain and suffering of apartheid South Africa, and although she was a powerful medicine woman who healed many from their ailments, she could not prevent her own heart condition, and the embedded grief that led to her sudden death. She did not get to see the end of apartheid, or get to vote in the first free election in South Africa, or get to see me, my sister, and my brother married and have children which was her dearest wish.

When I woke up this morning, I had a tight pain in my chest for a few seconds. I am exactly the same age today as Ellen was when she died just like that.

I reflect on the fact that even with all the tools and wisdom I have acquired through living this path of Ayurveda, I am bound to the ups and downs, the fluctuations in commitment to my own health, and the old habits which are so tempting to engage in. Those habits that numb out anxiety, emotional stress, and the unforeseen events of life.

It stops me in my tracks sometimes when I realize how short life can be and although I don't have control over life and death, I do have control over the choices I make, and how I wish to spend the time I do have here.

Today I choose to celebrate. I am grateful to be here. Happy birthday to me.

M

June 29th

Feeling so vata *vitiated. Staying up late, eating at irregular times, undertaking every form of* prajnaparadha *(crimes against wisdom) that there are. My Ayurvedic lifestyle has come to a screeching halt, and I don't care because I'm falling in love.*

Falling in love is certainly not practical, routine, or even sustainable, yet this magical time is precious, thrilling and exquisite. I wouldn't trade it for all of the kichari *in the world.*

I find myself feeling love so intensely, and concurrently watching the waves of doubt roll in to sabotage this ripening connection that I was yearning for. I asked for love, am ready for it, and still it hurts a little.

It's the pain of getting what I really want.

A wince in my eye at the beauty when it is right before my eyes, a shuddering through my body when he is here in my arms, and a piercing energy so intense that I cannot do anything but love this man with all of who I am despite circumstances being anything but perfect.

When is life ever the "perfect" that we imagine it should be? When perfect arrives in disguise, I honour and welcome it in my heart and resist it in the mind. Thankfully, my heart is wiser than my mind, and I trust in the feeling within. I pray for the strength to continually listen to the Grace within me that has always been guiding me home.

Chapter 20

Summer Routines

Seasonal and Daily Practices for Summer

After our Spring commitment to lighten up and clear out the old, we begin the Summer time with a sense of clarity and *joie de vivre*! The sun is out, and we are ready to play. Playtime, as George Bernard Shaw so simply put it, keeps us young. When we watch kids at play, it is a reminder of our own inner joy and light-hearted spirit, and we are uplifted.

Pitta dosha is activated in the Summer and flourishes with a cooling and regular self-care practice. Relaxed lunches, more time outdoors, spontaneous playtime, and slower activities that help to cool us down and avoid stress, all support a balanced Summer routine.

Funny how it is that it's easier to be spontaneous when we have a routine because we are taking care of business when we consistently take care of ourselves. It may take time and commitment to get into these feel good habits, but it makes such a huge difference to our well-being that we begin to crave them as part of our daily life.

Summer memories are always imbued with the outdoors, the sounds of the cicada, the sweet dry scent of the evenings, walks in the moonlight, camping under the stars, campfires, sipping Summer drinks on the deck, street fairs, festivals, mangos, watermelon, peaches, playing on the beach and swimming in the ocean. The list is infinite. Focus on relaxation and play by taking time out to enjoy the warmth and light and the lively, languorous joys of Summer.

Begin simply as always. Shift your practices to a more relaxed pace. Take a vacation, have a moonlight swim, eat a mango with your whole face, laugh, play, sleep outdoors, snorkel, ride a bicycle. The Summer daily practices will give you the footing to fly free and the stability to let loose. Sounds like a crazy contradiction?

Just put into place your Summer routine and you will find the downtime and spontaneous playtime available to you whenever you need it.

Gently get into a habit of waking a little earlier, by about 15 minutes. If you were waking in Spring at 6:45 a.m., you can slowly transition into waking at 6:30 a.m. and then at 6:15 a.m., or even 6 a.m. if you are aspiring to be a true morning bird. As always, allow yourself enough time to do your morning practices without feeling stressed or rushed.

1. Morning cleansing rituals: scrape tongue, brush teeth, start your oil pulling practice of swishing 1 tbsp coconut oil around inside the mouth. Coconut oil is cooling for the Summer and for *pitta dosha*.

2. Drink warm water with lime and a sprig of fresh mint. This will cool the body and mind, and activate your digestion for the day. You can also choose just mint, or just lime.

3. Massage coconut oil or ghee gently into both nostrils using either a cotton tip or your baby finger.

4. Beautiful Body and Happy Mind Summer Practices:

    - Meditate. (Even five minutes is a good start).

    - Breathe. Follow your Summer *pranayama* practice.

    - Move. (Follow your Summer yoga practice, dance, walk, swim, cycle, stretch). Cooler, slower movements help to prepare the body for the day without over exertion. An Ayurvedic philosophy is to exercise to half your capacity, which means you break a sweat and then you are done. No need to get into intense training for your self-care practice (unless you really are an athlete in training, but even then the Summer workouts can be cooler and slower). You can take your walks in the evening under the serene moonlight.

    - Self-massage with coconut oil will cool, nourish, and protect your skin. A regular self-massage practice relaxes the nervous system, removes impurities from the blood, and feeds the tissues of the body. Performing this even three times a week will bring lasting lifetime benefits.

    - Shower with an all natural gentle herbal soap to make you feel alive and bring vibrancy to your skin.

    - Anoint yourself with aromatic, sweet, and cooling essential oils. Choose from mint, sandalwood, rose, jasmine, geranium, vetiver, neroli, bergamot, lotus, ylang ylang, lavender, fennel, or coriander (see Summer self-care section for application).

5. Meals: Breakfast, lunch, and dinner taken at the same times each day will support a sense of calm and order—which *pitta* types crave and we all need—and also assists with good digestion. Fresh, light meals are ideal with a focus on bitter, sweet, and astringent tastes. Cooling herbs and spices keep the digestive fires burning without burning you up. Avoid oily, heavy foods such as fried foods, dense creamy soups, heavy grains, stews, and root vegetables. Salads with seeds, sprouts, and crunchy veggies are a perfect way to enjoy the bounty of the season. Eat away from the computer or other electronic distractions, perhaps outside or nearby an open window for fresh air.

    - Breakfast: Light and nourishing, eaten by 10 a.m.

- Lunch: Main meal of the day eaten around midday. Avoid over-eating. Take a short easy walk after lunch to aid digestion.

- Dinner: Light and freshly prepared, eaten ideally by 7 p.m. Avoid heavy foods in the evening as this can result in congestion and disturbed sleep with fiery violent dreams.

6. Before bed: Take some quiet time with at least an hour of distraction-free space. Meditate, journal, pray, chant, or write poetry. Choose an activity that integrates your day and brings a peaceful night sleep. Enough rest rejuvenates and relaxes the body and mind. Aim for bedtime between 10:30 p.m., and 11 p.m. (earlier if you can).

7. Generally, it is wise to avoid sleeping in the day, however in the Summertime, a short 10 minute, late afternoon nap in a hammock is delicious.

Engage in playfulness, silliness, and spontaneity—Summer is here!

Chapter 21

Summer Food Practices

Everything seems so much brighter in the Summer. Colors are intense and vibrant, fruits are juicy and sweet, and a playful mood is present in the air.

As our digestion is stronger in the Winter to keep our core warm, so it is weaker in the Summer as our *agni* is dispersed to the skin making us sweat to keep us cool. This is the hot season of the *pitta dosha*, and in Ayurveda, the food practices for this season are cool, light, and easy.

We also want to maintain balance and be sure not to accumulate toxins in the body by dousing our digestive fire with icy drinks and too cold foods. Understanding and applying this concept is the balance of Ayurveda and our guide to an easy, breezy Summer.

G

I nostalgically recall the sultry Summer nights growing up in Johannesburg surrounded by the sound of men shouting, "Heh Mielies." Mielies is the Afrikaans word for corn, and the taste of the Southern African corn mingling with the earthy scent of the African nights is indelibly imprinted on my taste bud memories.

Farmers would come with their wheelbarrows after dusk, walking through the suburban streets chanting their mielie mantra, multiple voices echoing in harmony. "Heh mielies, heh mielies, heh mielies".

We would run out of our houses waiting to see a mielie-barrow man so we could purchase big ears of this sweet Summer corn on the cob. The smell of butter melting on hot, sweet corn as we sank our teeth into the firm, juicy kernels is why I cannot do without my mielies in the Summer.

What happens to your body and mind in the Summer? After the Spring, the body may be somewhat phlegmatic if we have not observed our Spring cleansing rituals and daily routines. Early Summer colds result in a heaviness in the body and congestion in our lungs and upper respiratory system. This accumulation of *kapha*, mixed with Summer heat, may turn to uncomfortable swelling, excess heat, and sweating. If this excess water element left over from the Spring is not cleared, it can aggravate the fire/heat element in the body and start to show signs of imbalance through the skin. Rashes, irritation, heartburn, inflammation, acne, rosacea, and other heat/water related conditions can arise.

The focus in the Summer is to keep the body cool and the mind calm. We can set things right by shifting our diet and observing the Summer principles and practices for balance and well-being. This all happens through awareness. The qualities of the season are those akin to the fire and water elements like hot, oily, and pungent so we need to apply the Ayurvedic principles of opposites to regain balance.

The tastes to focus on at this time of year are bitter, sweet, and astringent.

Watch for the foods at your local market for clues to your seasonal diet. Summer fare abounds in bitter salad greens, bright yellow squash, zucchini, cooling cucumbers, fresh herbs and spices, and lighter grains. Basmati rice, couscous, barley, and tapioca are all abundant. As well, the good old fashioned corn-on-the-cob should *not* be ignored. Corn is heating and drying, and therefore not ideal for *pitta* types. However, when drizzled with ghee and eaten in combination with fresh salad greens, it is a treat on a hot Summer's eve for everybody.

> G
>
> *Sweet fruits are delicious and satisfying and make for less time in the kitchen and more time to play.*
>
> *I have fond memories of all the sweet juicy fruits being consumed in the hot South African Summers. I will never forget, nor have I found a replacement for, the yellow cling peaches, the guavas, the mangos, and the lychees.*
>
> *Having tasted such tropical southern fruits, I make an exception to buying only local fruits in the Summer. I must have my organic hairy mango, and my desire for watermelon and lychees must be satiated even if it comes from the generous bounty of another country far away.*

The intention for a balanced Summer food practice is sweet and easy, playful and exuberant.

Tip: Avoid hot, heavy, oily, spicy foods as they heat up the blood causing skin conditions, heat rashes, acid digestion, reflux, and inflammation. Avoid spicy pungent foods such as chilies, dry ginger, and excess black pepper. Summer burnout and overheating is aggravated by food and drink that creates acid and heat in the cardiovascular system, the liver and the blood. Avoid iced drinks and too much heavy, cold ice cream, as the digestive fire will be put out with excess cold.

Tonic: Sweet, bitter, and cooling tonics and teas are relaxing, delicious, and sustaining to body and mind! Enjoy teas of peppermint, lavender, rose, fennel, coriander, chamomile, and saffron. Take a quarter cup of aloe vera gel or juice in the morning before your breakfast, as this cools the system and lubricates the mucous membranes.

Treat: Delight in fruit smoothies by blending juicy fruits like mango with banana, hemp seeds, and coconut milk, or by blending watermelon, coconut water, lime, and fresh ginger juice.

Summer Food Guide

Herb and Spice Magic for the Summer

Aloe	Cilantro	Coriander	Cardamom	Cumin
Dill	Fennel	Ginger (fresh)	Mint	Orange Peel
Parsley	Rose Petals	Saffron	Spearmint	

Summer Legumes

Aduki Beans	Black Beans	Black-Eyed Peas	Chickpeas	Lentils (Green/Black)
Lima Beans	Navy Beans	Pinto Beans	Soybeans	Split Mung Beans
Split Peas	Tofu			

Summer Grains

Barley	Bulgur	Couscous	*Corn, fresh	Pasta (wheat, rice)
*Quinoa	Rice (white/basmati)	Spelt	Tapioca	Wheat
Unbleached white flour		Wheat Bran		

*In moderation

Summer Fruits

Apple (sweet)	Apricot (sweet)	Avocado	*Banana	Berries (sweet)
Coconut	Dates	Grapes	Guava	Lemon
Lime	Lychees	Mango	Melon	Orange (sweet)
Papaya (sweet)	Peaches	Plums (sweet)	Raisins	Watermelon

*In moderation

Summer Veggies

Acorn Squash	Artichoke	Arugula	Asparagus	Bell Peppers
Bok Choy	Broccoli	Celery	Cabbage	Cucumber
Daikon Radish	Endive	Green Beans	Jerusalem Artichoke	Jicama
Peas	Parsley	Salad Greens: Lettuce, Pea Shoots, Peppercress, etc.		
Seasonal Greens	Sprouted Seeds and Greens		Summer Squash	*Tomatoes

*In moderation

Summer Dairy

Cows Milk	Cottage Cheese	Ghee	Goats Cheese	Goats Milk
*Yoghurt, Naturally Sweetened				

*In moderation

Summer Fish and Meat

Chicken	Eggs	Fish (freshwater)
Shrimp	Turkey	Venison

Summer Seeds and Condiments

Coconut	Chutneys (fresh)	Flax Seeds
Hemp Seeds	Pumpkin Seeds	Sunflower Seeds

Avoid nuts in the Summer time as they are heating, oily, and heavy.

Summer Oils

Avocado	Canola	Coconut
Ghee	Olive	Sunflower

*In moderation

Summer Sweeteners

Barley Malt Syrup	Brown Rice Syrup	Dates	*Honey
Fruit Juice Concentrates		Maple Syrup	Cane Sugar (Raw, Unprocessed)

Summer Teas

Burdock Root	Coriander	Chamomile	Dandelion	Fennel
Mint	Rose petal	*CCF (Classic Ayurvedic tea of cumin, coriander and fennel)		

*To make CCF tea take 1 tsp each of fennel seed, cumin seed, and coriander seed. Add along with 4 cups water to a small pot and bring to boil. When mixture has reached a boil, turn down to simmer for 10-15 minutes. Strain and drink. This tea is cleansing, aids the digestive system and supports the absorption of nutrients in the body while bringing the body into a state of acid/alkaline (pH) balance. A great tea to reset the body after any over-indulgences.

Summer Meal Ideas and Recipes

Breakfast: Sweet, light grains such as basmati rice with coconut milk, sprinkled with saffron or fennel are a nourishing breakfast in the Summer. Add spices, seeds, herbs, and dried fruits from your Summer Food Guide for a satisfying meal to start your day off right.

- Sweet fruits melded as a fruit salad with a sprinkle of ground fennel, mint, and a squeeze of lime juice is a refreshing breakfast.

- Experiment with other seasonal grains, or try scrambled eggs with avocado and cucumber on toast.

- Try a yoghurt parfait with a berry compote sprinkled with hemp seeds.

- A smoothie with banana, coconut water, berries, and hemp seeds makes for a great morning booster.

Lunch: This is best as your main meal of the day as digestion is at its prime between noon and 2 p.m.

- Remember to include all six tastes for a balanced and satisfying meal.

- Light broths and raw salads with a variety of veggies, greens, and chickpeas are a delicious cooling lunch option.

- Summer greens, grains, beans, and small portions of animal foods make up a good lunch!

- Experiment with a variety of foods from the Summer Food Guide.

Dinner: This can be a lighter meal taken at least three hours before bedtime.

- Enjoy a variety of spices and condiments with your meal to include all six tastes.

- Soups, grains, small portions of animal foods, and a rotating variety of veggies is best.

- Simplicity is key for your daily evening meal. Focus on the bitter, sweet, and astringent tastes.

- Eat slowly, enjoy every bite.

- Offer gratitude before each meal.

Zesty Summer Gazpacho with a Twist

This quick and easy soup gives you more time to play!

Serves 4

2 cups water
1 cup coconut water
1 green bell pepper
1 head romaine lettuce
1 peeled cucumber
1 cup chopped parsley
1 cup chopped cilantro
4 tbsp sunflower seeds
1 tsp whole cane sugar
2 tsp lime juice
1 tsp cumin seeds toasted
2 large tomatoes diced
1 tbsp mint leaves
1 tsp salt

1. In a food processor or blender, mix together the water, coconut water, bell pepper, lettuce, peeled cucumber, parsley, cilantro, sunflower seeds and one tomato.

2. Blend ingredients until partially smooth so that you still maintain some texture. Add more water if needed.

3. Toast cumin seeds, and stir into blended soup along with the salt, sugar, and lime juice.

4. Mix in well.

5. Dice the one remaining tomato and mix with finely minced mint leaves, and lime juice. Mix together well and add a dollop to soup bowl when serving.

Enjoy this refreshing Summer soup with a hearty chunk of fresh whole grain bread of your choice slathered in ghee!

The Golden Ghee

Ghee is one of the most *sattvic* (pure and harmonizing) foods for the body. Making your own batch offers you both a peaceful meditation, as well as a magical healthy fat for cooking, for transporting herbs and healing foods into the system, and even for use as a topical moisturizer. Ghee is good for all *doshas* in the Summertime and is a specific tonic for *pitta*. Use daily for beautiful healthy skin, hair and nails.

Ghee keeps indefinitely without refrigeration, as the water element that causes butter to spoil has been removed in the cooking. Just remember to keep it covered and free from water or any other contaminants. Always dip into your ghee jar with a clean spoon.

Making your Ghee

You will need:

1lb unsalted, organic butter
Thick-bottomed stainless steel pot
Stainless steel spoon
Glass jar with secure lid

1. Sterilize the storage jar, pot and a spoon in advance by filling with (or immersing in) boiling water. Dry very well. Water in the ghee will contaminate it and make it go moldy.

2. Cook the butter gently over low heat for approximately 15-25 minutes.

3. Foam will form on the surface throughout the heating process. Scoop this off with a dry clean spoon as it collects. These are the milk solids. This can be put aside and used later for other purposes such as baking.

4. Watch carefully to avoid burning. Making ghee requires patience and awareness.

5. When the ghee begins to boil silently with only a trace of glassy air bubbles on the surface and a golden clear colour, it is ready. You should be able to see to the bottom of the pot without any sign of cloudiness.

6. Depending on the butter used, more milk solids may float on top. Strain off with a clean spoon.

7. Allow to cool and then pour ghee through a fine strainer or cheesecloth into the clean, dry glass container.

Super Duper Summer Smoothie

A great way to lighten up! Be adventurous and add your own health-giving extras.

1/2 cup of fresh or frozen blueberries, strawberries, raspberries, or blackberries
1 tsp spirulina powder (or other powdered chlorella/super greens)

1 cup coconut water
1 cup filtered water
1 tbsp almond butter
1/4 avocado
2 cups spinach, washed and roughly chopped
2 big leaves kale, washed and stems removed

Options to add for a sweeter smoothie:

1 tbsp cocoa powder (a bliss-inducing powerhouse full of antioxidants)
1 banana, frozen or fresh
2 tbsp hemp nuts

Add all ingredients together in a blender and blend until smooth and creamy.

A Sweet Summer Chutney

A delightfully zesty condiment.

2 sweet mangoes or peaches peeled and chopped
6 dates
1 cup boiling water to soak dates
1 tsp lime juice
1 tbsp fresh grated ginger
1 tsp raw cane sugar
1 tbsp desiccated coconut
1/4 tsp ground cardamom
5 strands saffron
Pinch of salt

1. Soak dates for 15 minutes in 1 cup boiled water while prepping fruits.

2. Remove pits from dates and save soaking water to add to mix.

3. In a food processor or blender, mix all ingredients until partially smooth, maintaining some of the texture. Add date soaking-water to your desired consistency.

4. May refrigerate for up to a week.

Use as a tangy condiment to sweeten and bring joy and celebration to your meals.

Summer Sleepy-time Sipper

To be taken half an hour before bed.

Add 3-5 strands of saffron and 1/8 tsp turmeric to 1/4 cup of warm milk.

Stir the saffron and turmeric into the warmed milk. Allow to cool to room temperature. You can add a small pinch of unrefined cane sugar to sweeten. Turmeric and saffron are both excellent purifying tonics for the blood and liver.

Chapter 22

Summer Self-Care Practices

The sun brings warmth and heat, which melts away inhibitions, stiffness, and heaviness. Summer is abundant in sweet juicy fruits that can be used as masks, tonics, and scrubs.

Our skin is in need of protection from the drying rays of the sun, as well as nourishment, to keep it moist, supple, and toned. Toes and feet are out and about and crave showing themselves off after being socked up in the cool, damp seasons.

Dropping rigid rules and having more playtime are the self-care elixirs for the season. Summer is time to pamper yourself with fabulous fun activities. So take off those socks, kick off your shoes, and let the tall green grass tickle your toes. Smile, laugh, howl at the moon, and salute the sun. Yes, Summer is here, and you deserve to enjoy it to the fullest.

After the Spring, when we have detoxed our liver and blood, we should find our skin glowing with health. Keeping it that way is the prime focus for the Summer season.

> G
>
> *I remember as a child growing up in the African Summer sun that one of my favourite experiences was watching and waiting for the watermelons bobbing up and down in our swimming pool to cool down, and then the excitement as we would jump in to choose one for our afternoon snack.*
>
> *Once it had been exploded open we would dive into it with glee, our whole face and body eating the watermelon, face dripping in sweet fresh juice.*
>
> *Afterwards, we would jump, sticky and happy, back into the pool to cool off and splash about.*

Watermelon makes a fantastic mask for all skin types because it is, of course, 93% water and loaded with vitamins such as A, B6, and C. This nourishes, hydrates, and repairs your skin from sun damage and guards against possible *pitta* blemishes.

Summer—being the *pitta* time of year—especially evokes the sense of sight. Cool and beautify your eyes with a cucumber compress sprayed lightly with rose water. Wash out your eyes weekly with cool, fresh, filtered water. Consider using apricot or coconut oil to thicken and add gloss to your lashes and eyebrows, rather than mascara, eyeliner, or eyebrow pencils. Drop a small amount of oil onto your fingertips, and gently oil the lashes in an upward motion being careful not to get any into your eyes.

Becoming aware of what you are taking in visually is also essential to healthy vision in a bigger sense. Our eyes are known as, "the mirror to our soul," connecting our outer and inner worlds. In Ayurveda the *pitta dosha*, being primarily the element of fire and light, governs our eyesight.

One of the five *pitta* fires known as *alochaka pitta* resides in our eyes absorbing and digesting images and in fact all visual impressions in our "technicolor" world. When this fire is in balance, our eyes glow with luminous health and look clear, bright, and shining.

For those who are a bit more adventurous, gazing at the sun is a *Vedic* practice that can improve eyesight. Bear in mind that solar gazing is only recommended at early dawn when the sun has just risen, or at dusk just as the sun is setting, so that harmful U.V. rays cannot injure the eyes. One can gently gaze at the sun starting with 10 seconds, and increasing time by 10 second increments daily up to one minute.

Of course the best beauty tip is a good nights rest. Avoiding going to bed after 11 p.m. is the best way to keep eyes sparkly, and to restore the body. In the Summer, with its longer days, it is tempting to go to bed well into the fiery *pitta* time of night. This, however, may lead to burnout, exhaustion, and puffy red eyes.

Here are some simple self-care practices which will tickle your fancy and make you feel pretty, free, and happy all season long.

Happy Summer Face Polish

Make a one or two week supply of this protective cleanser for glowing skin. Use in the morning to cleanse your face.

Dry ingredients

1 cup finely ground basmati rice
1/4 cup dried ground rose petals
1 tsp dried and finely desiccated coconut (unsweetened)
1 tsp finely crushed dried mint
(Blend together, store in an airtight glass jar in a cool dry place or in the refrigerator)

Wet ingredients

Water, coconut water, or rose water
(Keep separate, and add to dry mix to make into a paste for each cleansing application)

For your daily morning face cleansing ritual:

1. Take a tbsp of the dry mixture and add enough water or coconut water or rose water to make into a creamy thick consistency.
2. Mix into a paste and with upward sweeping and circular strokes massage over entire neck and face.
3. Add more liquid if necessary to get a smooth application.
4. Without scrubbing, gently massage face all over with this light and cooling nutrient-rich cleanser for your vibrant Summer skin.
5. Wash off with cool water, and gently pat skin dry with a clean towel.

Summer Face Shield

Protect your skin from sun and the elements of fire with a light cooling moisturizer. After cleansing, use this in the morning to replenish and brighten your skin for the day.

1 cup unrefined coconut oil
1 tsp vitamin E oil (optional)
1 tsp rosehip oil
12 drops peppermint EO
6 drops rose geranium EO
3 drops sandalwood or lavender EO
1 bottle rose water or witch hazel toner to have on hand (do not mix into blend until using)

Mix rosehip, coconut, and vitamin E oil together along with the essential oils. Store in an airtight glass bottle.

Each morning after cleansing, take 1/4 tsp (a few drops) of oil blend and mix with 1/2 tsp witch hazel toner or rose water. Massage into face with upward circular strokes.

Summer Face Slushie

A weekly face mask will keep your skin bright, cool, and glowing and protect it from oily blemishes and the harsh rays of the sun.

1/2 cup watermelon pulp
1 tbsp aloe vera gel (whole leaf or inner fillet)
1 tbsp whole milk plain yoghurt
3 drops geranium, rose, or lavender essential oil.

Mix together and apply generously to face. Lie in your hammock, outside on your deck, or in a cool place inside. Leave on for 10-15 minutes. Wash off with cool water. Glowing skin!

Summer Foot Relief and All Over Body Cooler

You will not believe how great this foot treatment and body chiller feels. If your feet are hot, sweaty, and achy take one of these icy cubes and apply. Also great for sunburn and hot, sun-kissed skin.

2 cups water
1 cup mint leaves
1/4 cup rose water or coconut water
Juice from one lime

Mix the fresh mint, water, rose water or coconut water and lime juice together and add to blender. Add to ice cube trays and stick in the freezer. Take one out when you are feeling hot and bothered and want a tantalizing skin refresher.

Summer Aromatherapy

Every season brings an opportunity to make friends with the healing plant essences. We may use essential oils to balance the hot, oily, intense qualities of the season that can affect our body and make us feel burned out, irritated, and overheated. A simple single note oil or a blend of any of the Summer oils can keep your emotions cool and relaxed and your body fragrant and sweet. Wherever I go, people always tell me how lovely I smell. I never go a day without using my essential oils.

Slowly build your aromatherapy apothecary for each season and you will always have a remedy on hand. The oils are versatile and can be blended in a multitude of ways.

Suggested Essential Oil List for Summer
(Cooling, soothing, restorative, sweet, easy, simple)

Stock your bathroom apothecary with at least three or four of these fragrant friends:

mint, sandalwood, rose, jasmine, geranium, vetiver, neroli, eucalyptus, rosewood, patchouli, lavender, ylang ylang, artemisia (mugwort).

How to apply aromatherapy to your daily Summer practice:

Make a pure essential oil blend using two or three different oils. Store in a dark glass airtight bottle. You can also keep four or five different essential oils in your bathroom cabinet and blend as needed or use individually as preferred.

1. Massage oil: By adding an essential oil blend to a carrier oil you can have a customized massage blend on hand to use. Two lovely massage carrier oils for the Summer are coconut or grapeseed oil (or an equal mix of the two). A ratio of between 48-90 drops of pure essential oil to 4 oz carrier oil is the standard range depending on how potent you want your blend. Keep your blend simple when starting out using only three or four essential oils. Play and experiment as you discover the best scents for you.

2. Bath oil: The best way to use essential oils in the bath is to mix them with salts or an emulsifier such as fresh milk or your carrier oil. A good ratio is 10-20 drops essential oil, mixed with 1/2 cup of salt or emulsifier.

   You can also add your custom massage blend directly into the bath. 2-3 tbsps will make for a luxurious bath and will allow the oils to be absorbed deeply into the skin.

   Aromatic baths in the Summer are excellent for the endocrine and adrenal systems, and for restoring the body-mind from burnout arising from excessive exertion.

3. Direct Palm Inhalation: Apply 1-2 drops of essential oil to the palms, rub together gently, and inhale deeply. This is an excellent method for a quick and easy exposure to the essential oils.

4. Facial splash: 1-3 drops essential oil in cool water in a bowl or basin. Splash face with cooling, aromatic water. This mixture can also be used for spraying the face when irritable or overheated.

G & M's Summer Journals

G

July 25th

Today I visited the Vancouver Art Gallery for the first time in ages. As I walked around it seemed that colours exploded off the walls like urgent messengers, telling me in a language I understood to go get some canvases and pull out my brushes and paint. To go and create art for art's sake.

Soon after I returned home full of ideas and enthusiasm, my critical mind took over and replaced my desire for creating with the unwelcome din of doubt. There are always reasons not to respond freely to the creative yearnings of the soul: life is too busy, there are more important things to do, too tired, paints packed away deep in the storage closet, and a million other reasons. None of these seem good enough.

I allowed the doubt to take over, completely quelling my energy and desire to paint. The usual dilemma cropped up of how best to spend my time when I feel I have so little of it to spare.

I have built my healing massage practice, my aromatherapy business, and grown my position as a teacher and writer through passion, dogged determination, and a deep desire to be above all, true to my calling and to give to others. Sometimes I feel I should just choose one thing and simplify but I am too greedy at the banquet of life. I pray for one of those thunderbolt, hit-by-lightning, shaktipat* *moments where suddenly all is clear. A revelation, a life transforming awakening that happens to those who are available to receive this grace at a time of confusion. I yearn for that clarity, that instantaneous gift of aha!*

I know when I feel this way there is nothing to do, nothing to decide. I calm down and consider where I am in my life and see that everything is as it should be. I understand having been here before in this place of overwhelm that I only need to continue to deepen my usual practices and to continue to transform my inner environment.

And to simply be.

* Shaktipat *is the conferring of spiritual "energy" upon one person by another and can be transmitted with a sacred word or mantra, or by a look, thought or touch usually to the* ajna chakra *or third eye of the recipient.*

Shaktipat *is also considered an act of grace on the part of the guru or the divine so you can see things about yourself and others more clearly and with more awareness.*

M

July 16th

One month in India. It was a journey of completion cloaked in the guise of taking students to an ashram to experience the "roots" of Yoga. India, and what it has offered me over the last 12 years, has been enormous: insight, my Guru, a spiritual name, initiation into an ancient lineage, connection to a spiritual community, and a land with such varied experiences, from the most expansive and enlightening Masters to the dirtiest toilets and dysentery (and everything in between). I am grateful for all of this as I would not be who I am today without these experiences, and I am ready to shed my identity and attachment to all of it. Not in a resentful way, but in a way that is connected to a deeper aspect of myself, the part that knows when something is complete.

So what is complete?

A cycle. Karma. *My need to look, act, feel or be a certain way because I think that who I am is a Yoga teacher. Who I am is Divine (as we all are), and in a subtle and sneaky way the truth of my essence has been masked by my identity as a "spiritual aspirant." The irony is that my Spirit has been stunted, knocked down and kept small by trying to be something that I already am . . . Whole. Complete. Perfect. Spiritual. Divine. Accepted. Loved. Free.*

Freedom is not in the searching or collecting of knowledge, wisdom, teachers or experiences.

Freedom can only be found in this present moment,
this perfect moment in the here and now . . .
and now . . .
and now . . .
and now . . .

Chapter 23

Summer Yoga, *Pranayama,* and Meditation Practices

Yoga. Oh Yeah!

In the brightness and heat of Summer, use your yoga practice to bring balance by cooling down and relaxing your body and mind.

Reduce excess *pitta* through your daily yoga practice by moving calmly, slowly, and in a non-competitive way through the postures.

Focus on the being rather then the doing.

Dissolve any idea of getting something out of your practice and focus on the joy of being present in the moment, without a result-driven motivation.

> **Summer Flow Tips**
>
> ~ Be consistent.
> ~ Generate routine by practicing at the same time everyday.
> ~ The ideal time to practice: early mornings or in the cool evening.
> ~ Manage your energy by noticing where it is going; increase your energy with a non-competitive and non-judgemental approach.
> ~ Remember you are perfect as you are right now!

Yoga Time

During the Summer months you may naturally find yourself with more energy as we get more *prana* from the strength and vitality of the Sun's power. If you've got a propensity towards doing more rather than less, pushing through rather than resting, then this sequence is dedicated to you—and equally appropriate for all during the heat of the *pitta* time of year—to bring balance during the extroverted energy of the season.

An Ayurvedic yoga practice in the Summer season brings balance by focusing on relaxing, cooling, and calming your energy through an effortless, non-competitive approach using slow and steady movement as well as stillness, to accentuate the importance of non-doing or better known as being.

The home site of *pitta dosha* is in the small intestine: Therefore, postures that massage, focus on, and draw attention here cool an overheated *pitta* individual.

If you find yourself being irritated easily, yelling like a madwoman at the postman, or giving people the finger while driving, please follow this yoga class.

Twists are some of the best postures to pacify the overheated and intense *pitta*, as are postures that stimulate the liver, detoxify the blood, and cleanse the mind, reminding *pitta* personalities that all is perfect now.

No, really, *everything is perfect* . . .

Maybe things are not the way you want them to be, but there is a sweet perfection that the Universe has served up in the take-out container of your life. Eat it up, digest it with gratitude, and eliminate what is not providing you with a nutritious, joyful, and vibrant life.

This practice is short and succinct and can be done in 20 minutes.

1. Howz Those Hips? (*Baddha Konasana*: Bound Angle)
(1 min.)

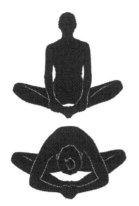

Sit on the floor with your knees bent and out to the sides so that the soles of your feet are touching. If your lower back is slumped, sit on a yoga block or folded up blanket to give a little bit of height. Hold onto your ankles. Inhale; elongate your spine. Exhale, hinge forward from your hips, allowing your heart to melt towards the earth. Relax here, and breathe for 5-10 breaths.

2. The Cat's Meow (*Marjariasana*: Cat Stretch)
(1 min.)

Come up onto your hands and knees. Place your shoulders directly above your wrists and your hips directly above your knees. Spread your finger bones open like fans and press the entire surface of your hand into the floor. Inhale—begin by tipping your tailbone towards the sky and dipping your abdomen towards the earth. Continue to sequence through the spine until your chest and gaze are also looking upwards (if you are feeling overheated, keep your gaze at the floor so that your head doesn't lift as high). Exhale—draw your tailbone down to point towards the ground as you lift your navel up towards the ceiling, dropping the head to the chest. Repeat 5 times.

3. Child's Pose...Aaaaawh (*Balasana*: Pose of the Child)
(1 min.)

Press your buttocks back to sit on your heels, resting your forehead on the ground (if your buttocks do not rest on your heels, place a pillow or folded blanket in between them so that you can relax). Bring your arms by your sides, palms upwards with the elbows slightly bent. Breathe slowly and deeply into the belly 5-10 times.

4. Fly! Fly! Fly Away! (*Salabhasana*: Locust)
(2 min.)

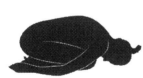

Come down so that you are on your belly with your legs straight out behind you and your arms down by your sides. On your next inhalation, lift your legs, chest, arms, and head off of the floor. Keep your gaze down at the ground in front of you. Stay here and breathe for 5 deep breaths in and out. Come back down to the starting position on an exhalation.

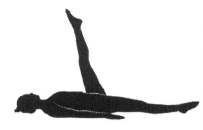

5. Leg Lifts for Life
(2 min.)
Lying on your back with your legs together and palms by your sides facing down, relax your entire body into the floor. Inhale—lift your right leg up to a 90 degree angle. Exhale, slowly lower the leg back down. Repeat with the left leg. Alternate the leg lifts until you have done 5 with each leg. Stage two of the practice is to inhale and lift the right leg while simultaneously raising the left arm. Exhale and lower the right leg and left arm at the same time towards the floor. Repeat on the second side, lifting the left leg and right arm up to 90 degrees on the inhalation and slowly lowering on the exhalation. Do a total of 5 rounds of stage two on both sides.

6. The "Grande Schebang": Hip Opener (*Kapotasana*: Pigeon)
(3 min.)
Begin by coming onto all fours or "downward dog". Gently place your right knee on the floor to the inside of your right hand. Bring the pelvis forward and down, keeping the weight evenly distributed between both sides of your pelvis. The left leg is straight out behind the left hip with the top of the foot facing the floor. Inhale—lengthen your spine, exhale and allow your torso to elongate and lower towards the earth. You may like to stay upright with weight on your hands, come onto your forearms, or lower your forehead onto two stacked fists. Stay for 5-10 breaths. Relax and focus on the exhale, on letting go. Slowly come back out of the posture on an inhalation. Press your hands into the ground, lift the weight of your pelvis up and transition through "downward facing dog" posture before going to the second side.

If you experience any pain in your knee or hip, this posture is not for you.

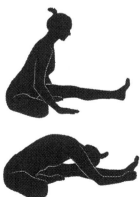

7. Grade 10 Gym Class (*Janu Sirsasana*: Head to Knee)
(2 min.)
Sit on the ground with your legs straight out in front of you. Bend your right knee in towards your chest with the foot on the floor. Open the knee out to the right side (you may place your right foot on your thigh if your hips are really flexible). If your knee doesn't come close to the floor, support it with a yoga block or rolled up blanket. Inhale—lengthen your spine, exhale and relax your torso over the extended leg. Focus more on keeping your spine long rather than getting your head close to your extended leg. Stay for 5 breaths. Inhale to return upright. Bring your right leg back together with the left. Repeat on the left side. Take one inhalation here.

8. Twistin' Round (*Ardha Matsyendrasana*: Seated twist)
(2 min.)

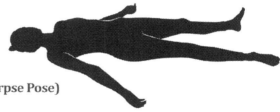

While sitting with both of your legs extended in front of you, bend your right knee, place your right foot on the floor on the outside of your left leg. If you have the flexibility, bend your left knee and tuck your left heel in towards your left sitting bone, otherwise keep your left leg straight. Inhale—lengthen your spine, hug the outside of your right leg with your left arm, place your right hand on the floor behind you. Exhale—twist your torso to the right, drawing your right leg in towards your body (this naturally massages your internal organs). Turn your head to look at the wall behind you without strain. Stay for 5 breaths. Inhale to return to centre, release the legs and prepare for the second side.

9. Icing on the Cake (*Savasana*: Corpse Pose)
(5-7 min.)

Savasana is your time to be still and quiet. No planning, fixing, or sorting through your to-do list in your mind. Surrender. Acceptance. Patience. Release your body weight to the support of the earth beneath you. Accept your current state of body and mind, and be patient for the unfolding of your life so that it is graceful, organic, and fluid. Indulge in your relaxation practice for 5-7 minutes.

Lay down on your back with your head and spine straight, legs apart, letting the feet flop out to the sides. Arms are away from the sides of the body slightly, and the palms face upward. Close your eyes.

Let your entire body relax. Begin at your toes and relax your feet. Move your awareness up through the body all the way to the head, consciously letting go of any stress or tension along the way. Your breath should be completely natural. Surrender into the stillness and silence of this posture.

Once you have completed the practice, start to wiggle your fingers and toes. Stretch your body in any way that feels great!

Roll to one side, and use your hands to push yourself to an upright position.

Honour Yourself

Take a moment to observe how you are feeling physically, mentally, emotionally, and energetically after your yoga practice.

Thank yourself for doing the practice (gratitude expands more of what we want in our life).

Honour your strengths and weaknesses (for the lessons you learn from them) of mind and body. Acceptance goes a long way.

Summer *Pranayama*: Cool It

It is quite easy to be continually amazed by the miraculous built-in power of our bodies. We are programmed with all of the operating systems that we need to adapt to a myriad of life situations and, most importantly, for survival.

Most of us have no idea about the treasure chest of goodies right here in our own body. You can heat up or cool down your body through these simple ancient *pranayama* practices.

Use the effective breathing practice of *sheetali* to cool your body temperature, chill heated emotions, pacify hot flashes, balance hormones, and relax yourself when your fuses are burning out.

The How-To of *Sheetali* Breathing

1. Sit in a comfortable position (in a chair, with your back against the wall, or crossed legged)—wherever you can have an elongated spine.
2. Establish a slow, calm, and steady breathing pattern in and out of your nostrils.
3. Stick out your tongue and curl the edges of your tongue to create a tube. Take a long, slow, steady breath in through the tongue. Focus on this cooling air entering the body.
4. At the end of your inhalation, close your mouth and exhale through the nose.
5. Repeat 10-50 times.

Practice Tips

- If you feel light-headed at any time, take a break.

- If you are unable to curl your tongue like a tube then open your mouth really wide, but keep your teeth together. Inhale the breath through the teeth, and follow the above directions.

Madhuri Phillips and Glynnis Osher

Summer Meditation: Laughing Towards Ecstasy

We have all heard that laughter is the best medicine. So why don't we take this free and easy medicine daily?

With adulthood there seems to be a looming heaviness equated with responsibility, maturity, and what it means to be "grown up." Some of the most enlightened people you could ever meet on this planet exude the sheer lightness and playfulness of a child. They are seemingly free from the burdens that the rest of us certainly thought were part of our rites of passage into adulthood: paying bills, covering rent, ever bettering ourselves, daily stress.

What we come to realize is that stress has little to do with the external situation or circumstance but more to do with an internal wiring, belief, or feeling about our relationship to a situation or circumstance. That is why two people can go through almost identical life traumas and either use the situation for their elevation or allow it to smother them completely.

Laughing is one of the best ways to release stress in the mind and body, decrease the risk of heart problems, and boost immunity. Laughter *really is* good medicine. Think of all of the different kinds of laughter; the cackle, crying laugh, thigh slapper, giggle, guffaw, chuckle, nervous laugh, snort, or, a personal favourite, laughing so hard that nothing comes out . . . the silent laugh!

Laughter helps to cool the fiery nature of the *pitta* individual and helps them not to take themselves or life too seriously. Laughter is as important as work, and facilitates the maintenance of good health and happiness. There are so many ways to tap into the brightness and friskiness of laughter to lift your spirits:

- Try the laughter meditation below.

- Watch a funny movie or TV show (Mr. Bean, John Cleese, Mike Myers, Steve Carell).

- Hang out with funny people.

- Read funny comics and/or books.

- Play fun games with friends (charades, go bowling, sing karaoke).

- Spend time with children and you will laugh, laugh, laugh!

- Dress up in a funny costume/ do something out of the ordinary or out of your comfort zone.

The How-To of the Laughing Meditation

1. It may seem obvious, but you do not need to have something to laugh at to begin laughing. Just do it. The motto here is fake it until... it happens. If that currently seems impossible then:

2. Lift your hands up towards the sky, look up and begin to laugh out loud with a forced "ha ha ha ha" for at least a minute.

3. Clap your hands strongly in front of your heart, laugh out loud, "ho ho ho ho."

4. Place your hands on your chest and laugh: "ha ha ha."

5. Switch between laughing—"ho ho ha ha ho ho."

6. Put your hands on the top of your head and laugh: "hee hee hee."

7. Stomp the floor and laugh—"hu hu hu."

8. Bend forward from the waist, let your arms hang; raise your torso and arms into the air while laughing like a hyena.

9. If you are still not laughing, go to the Doctor to make sure you have a pulse!

Meditation Tips

- The body cannot discern between true laughter and fake laughter, it has the same physiological and psychological impact.

- So go on, and giggle away!

Chapter 24

Summer Ceremony and Ritual

Think of childhood campfires and how the Summer is so carefree out in Nature under the brightly shining stars. There is something about the vivid, bold flames and the leaping spears of fire that open us up to singing, storytelling, and sharing our hearts with carefree abandon. When we think about it now, it makes sense that the feelings of aliveness and freedom are related to the transformative fire itself.

Summertime is a powerful time of transition, as the Summer Solstice is an astronomical solar event that marks the beginning of the season of fire and light. We benefit from the intensity of this season by burning up any leftover, deep-seated fears and obstacles. We build our courage, fortified by the solar energy. The actions of the stars and planets affect us deeply as does the changing of the seasons.

Many cultures around the world celebrate the solstice by building a huge community bonfire and throwing offerings into the blaze. These gifts to the fire take many forms. Some could say they are symbolically throwing themselves into the fire to transform and purify their intentions and purpose in this life, and to elevate their awareness. Others would offer up their darkest secrets, their perceived failures, and their fears, and let the power of the fire burn away these obstacles.

The element of fire serves to enlighten, to lighten up, and to transform so you are truly free. Setting up your altar on the solstice is a powerful affirmation of your choice to align with your true purpose, and your most vibrant health, transforming old limiting habits into new expansive ones.

Another fire ritual akin to the bonfire is called *Agnihotra* (*agni* means fire, *hotra* means healing). This is an ancient fire ceremony that comes from India's *Vedas*. The *Vedas* are some of the oldest sacred texts or scriptures of knowledge ever written, said to be channeled from cosmic consciousness.

These fire ceremonies were used to heal mental, emotional, physical, and karmic obstacles. They were used to harness the intelligence and transformative power of the fire element to shift awareness, resolve inner turmoil, burn up doubt, fear, negativity, and reveal inner light.

These Summer rituals are prescribed for transformation:

- To shift our awareness to joy and truth.
- To elevate our perception of our purpose.

- To celebrate playful light energy.
- To create our life of powerful abundance.
- To allow our rising up from the ashes so we can manifest our magnificent potential.

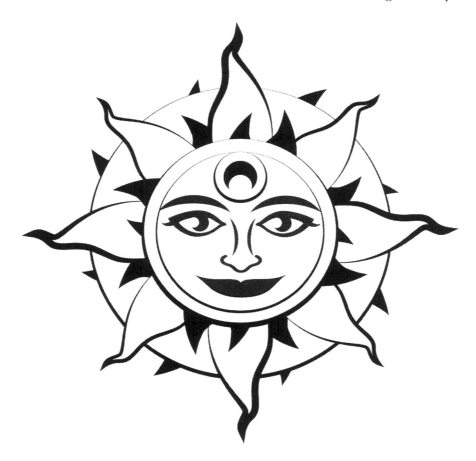

Summer Ceremony Themes: Light, Fire, Transformation, Play

Create your Summer sacred space: bright flowers, candles, playful objects, quotes from leaders or authors who inspire you, symbols of the Sun.

Remove all of the Spring objects from your altar and place a new brightly coloured cloth—or covering and other meaningful items—to mark the season.

Summer rituals remind us of our courage, our commitment, our profound light of intelligence, and our playful nature. Energized by the Summer Solstice, our ritual is powered by the Sun burning off our doubts, fears, and resistance to growth.

This is a seasonal opportunity to further refine and lighten your load, bringing you to your highest personal goals.

What you will need to create your own symbolic bonfire or fire ceremony:

1. Large sheet of paper for your Summer vision board. You can use white or a brightly coloured paper like yellow or orange.

2. Crayons, markers, tape, chalk, pencils, paint, glue, magazines.

    - Using the provided visual template as a guide, create your own symbolic fire ceremony. Draw or collage your personal bonfire on paper leaving room on either side of the symbol for pasting or writing words. You can use the symbol of the Sun or flames as your centerpiece. Let your playful creativity guide you.

    - Whenever you are inspired to do so, write a word or sentence on the left side of your fire symbol reflecting something that you feel is holding you back, bringing you pain, or that you wish to release—something you wish to burn up and transform in your fire ceremony. Some examples would be "scared of failure," or "unfit and sluggish," or "unlovable."

    - On the right side of the page coming out of the fire write or stick words or images that describe how you intend or want to feel. Such as—confident, beautiful, fit, playful, grounded, lovable, and irresistible.

You may find the actual words themselves have overlapped so much that they have become part of the centre symbol having been consumed and transformed by the fire of your intention and commitment.

Feel free to use this fire mandala template for your guide or create your own!

As a sacred environment that is set up and energized with your intentions, your altar acts as the witness, holding the space for your ceremonies and rituals. Once you have set up your personal space for ritual you may find that small miracles begin to happen.

Awakenings may spark new ideas, feelings of joy, and motivation. If you have not already set up your altar space, now is an optimal time to do so.

Chapter 25

7-Day Easy Juicy Summer Cleanse

Why a Summer Cleanse?

When the heat of the season sets in, the *pitta dosha* becomes vulnerable and various health issues can arise if not addressed. Flushing the liver and blood in the hot months by following a cooling and reducing diet can keep your body in an excellent state of health. Imbalance may show up as infections, inflammation, hyperacidity, bad breath and body odor, and excessive sweating.

As your complexion is a reflection of your inner health, acne, rashes, breakouts, and skin inflammations may also indicate toxic overload in the system. To prevent these symptoms, give your digestion a break and assist your body by lightening up.

A Summer cleanse is a joy as it includes fresh fruit and veggie juicing, smoothies made from nutrient-rich nuts, seeds, berries, and salads with cardio-protective and antioxidant rich oils like olive, avocado, flax, and coconut oil dressings with a ceremonial squeeze of lime. Including such foods into your Summer Cleanse brings extraordinary superwoman-like energy as well as clarity and lightness of body and mind. Yeah!

A 7-Day Summer Cleanse can be just the thing you need to glow. In Ayurveda, it is said that in 7 days we can turn our health around. Try it!

This is *not* a fast. It is a revitalizing light diet for a short duration to give you vitality so you can sparkle inside and out. Juices replenish electrolytes—the minerals we lose through the excess sweating we experience in the Summer. So, turn your fridge into a salad and smoothie bar.

Do not go hungry.

Enjoy the Benefits of a Summer Cleanse

- Improved digestion
- Radiant clear skin
- More energy and strength
- Better sleep
- Healthy weight
- Mental peace and clarity
- Improved attitude
- Increased levels of playfulness
- Juicy, JUICY you!

Shopping list for everything you need:

- Sweet, juicy fruits (seasonal)
- Salad greens (organic when possible)
- A rainbow variety of salad veggies (seasonal)
- Coconut water
- Coconut milk
- Aloe vera gel or juice
- Spices and herbs: coriander, cumin, fennel, turmeric, parsley, cilantro, dandelion, mint.
- Seeds and nuts: hemp nuts, coconut, sunflower seeds, blanched/soaked and peeled almonds (in moderation)
- *Triphala*
- Spirulina (powdered)
- Herbal teas: Choose a variety of cooling cleansing seasonal teas such as peppermint, dandelion, fennel, neem, and rose.
- Coconut oil (for self-massage)

Cleanse Prep:

Prep your salad and juice bar ingredients. Slice bell peppers, slither cucumbers, chop apples, strip lettuce. Keep chunks of ready-to-eat watermelon, melon, peaches, and other sweet juicy fruits in the fridge. Stock up on coconut water, fresh young coconuts, bitter greens, and sunflower seeds.

Your Summer Cleanse Calendar

Each Day:

- Scrape your tongue.
- Take aloe vera gel, an Ayurvedic panacea for Summer digestion and cleansing.
- Practice daily self-massage with coconut or sunflower oil or a blend of the two.
- Incorporate the Summer yoga practice into your day.
- Consume enough water, green juices, and herbal teas.
- Do your daily Summer *pranayama* practice.
- Commit to your Summer meditation practice.

Days 1-2

Introduce cooling herbal teas to flush heat from the organs. Choose from dandelion, fennel, mint, chamomile, or neem.

Day 1:

- Eliminate dairy, alcohol, caffeine, chocolate, sugar, animal products, processed foods, and sodas. This will be for the duration of the cleanse.

- Begin taking 1/4 cup aloe vera gel in the morning before eating.

- Make at least one meal on Day 1 a raw food meal. Make a super salad with a variety of greens and chopped veggies. Avoid broccoli and other veggies that are hard for you to digest when raw. Use a simple dressing of lemon juice and sunflower oil with a pinch of salt. Use fresh chopped herbs for flavouring your dressing: cilantro, arugula, watercress, parsley, dill, mint.

Day 2: Same as Day 1.

Days 3-6

You start to lighten and free the body from excess heat and acidity by enjoying the delicious fruits and veggies of the season in their nutrient-rich raw form. Drink fresh cool (not cold) filtered water when thirsty. Be sure to stay hydrated and flush toxins from the body by drinking enough water throughout the day. You'll find a Super Duper Summer Smoothie recipe to use as a guide in the Summer Meal Ideas and Recipes.

Day 3: All meals will be raw salads and/or smoothies. Adorn your salads with herbs, spices, and seeds. Vary your veggies. Add avocado to your salads for richness. Blend hemp nuts or sunflower seeds into your smoothies for extra strength. Add spirulina as a powerhouse antioxidant.

Day 4: Same as Day 3. If you have a juicer, juice bitter greens with sweet apples, cucumber, and lime for an afternoon pick-me-up.

Day 5: Same as Day 3 and 4. Experiment with the smoothie recipe. Add a sweet, ripe banana for a yummy-delish breakfast.

Day 6: Same as Day 3, 4 and 5. Smoothies, juices, salads . . .

Day 7

As with any cleanse, coming out of it is as important as the cleanse itself.

This is the last day of your Summer cleanse. Same as Days 3-6 with the addition of incorporating light grains into your diet.

Slowly over the next few days begin to reintroduce a variety of light grains, healthy proteins (nuts, legumes, eggs), fruits (eaten separately from other foods), and vegetables. Refer to the Summer food lists for guidance.

Daily Cleanse Check-in

Day	How do you feel today? Physically, mentally, emotionally?	What is your energy level like today? (from 1, lowest, to 10, highest)	What challenges are you currently experiencing?
1			
2			
3			
4			
5			
6			
7			

Keep doing your daily practices to support you through your 7-Day Summer Cleanse.

Part 5

Fall Time

Chapter 26

The Abundance of Fall

"Ring the bells that can still ring. Forget your perfect offering. There is a crack in everything, that's how the light gets in."

~ Leonard Cohen

M

I have always relished the Autumn time, particularly the transition from the extended sun-kissed days of Summer into the colourful crisp, fresh days of Fall. Memories abound of skipping rope, crunching leaves under my shoes, and playing Kick the Can in the backyard with the neighbourhood kids in an attempt to stretch out the final days of Summer as long as we could.

My birthday always fell within the first week of school. It really was a rebirthing, a time to start fresh. Clothes were cleaned and pencils were sharpened as we headed back to school. Every year, there was a maturing that seemed to take place over the Summertime which prepared me for another year.

In that first week off the beach and back sitting at the desk, there was something so satisfying about cracking open an untouched notebook in order to draw the title page. For me, those initial writings were symbolic of new beginnings and creation, as they foreshadowed what knowledge, wisdom, and growth would percolate behind the cover page of that book for the entire year.

The Autumn still carries this essence for me. Change. Transformation. A time to reassess and regroup: It's harvest time! As this is going on internally, Nature is expressing these sentiments externally with the leaves changing colours and drying up, the air cooling off and nipping at our noses, and birds beginning to migrate south for a relaxing holiday in Florida.

Ayurvedically speaking, the Fall is characterized and amplified by the qualities of change, cold, light, dry, clear, rough, and mobile. These qualities are related to *vata dosha*. In Fall, welcome in *vata's* opposite qualities to bring balance to your life. Think warm soups and stews, a woolen scarf around your neck and hat to cover your ears, daily relaxation, meditation, and routine, routine, routine.

During this time of year, we can easily find our selves spinning, tumbling, spiraling out of control with an over-active mind, feeling uber-stressed, overwhelmed, and maybe even a little bit crazy.

Been there?

Worry not, this is simply your *vata* out of balance, along with an over-taxed nervous system. By following a few cardinal suggestions (we don't like to use "rules" in Ayurveda), you can turn your Fall frenzy into Fall freedom.

8 Fall Journal Questions

1. What does the Fall season represent to you?
2. What qualities are invoked within you during the Fall season?
3. What you love about the Fall time is . . .
4. What three things can you do for yourself this Fall season to stay balanced physically, mentally, and emotionally?
5. Where would you like to direct your energy this season?
6. How can you do that?
7. What aspect of yourself is no longer serving you that you are ready to evolve out of?
8. What aspect of yourself would you like to expand?

G & M's Fall Journals

G

September 20th

I notice the refreshing feeling that comes from having taken nine hours sleep last night. I sometimes feel a bit guilty doing this. I am somewhat of a workaholic. Ever since art school in my late teens, I have stayed up into the wee hours creating. I always had school, a part-time job and several projects on the go at the same time. And then later, I had an intense 12-15 hours a day job in advertising, a small children's clothing company on the side, my yoga practice, and busy life in New York City. I have always been ambitious and filled with vision and passion and the feeling that life is never going to be long enough for me to accomplish everything I came here to do. How can I execute every idea, tell every story, pursue every education opportunity, see the world, change the world and spend time with friends and family and fit in my Ayurvedic practices?

I have of late become much wiser about how I spend my time. Rather than fighting my nature to fit in all the routines prescribed by the wisdom of Ayurveda, I engage in the ones that make sense with who I am. And I give myself a no-rules-day every week. This gives my pitta *mind a diversion and an escape route. I can eat, do or not do anything I want that day. It's like a day off for everything. Judgement and guilt are not invited.*

Well it turns out I have come to a place where my practices have begun to make more space rather than take more space in my life. How is this possible? I am still the busy multi-armed, multi-tasking, mighty manifesting miracle maker that I always was.

What happened is: consistent morning walks around the lake, my daily anointing and body oiling, my beloved's morning kisses, and my joyful spirit that now seems to have declared itself boss.

M

October 5th

For most of my life I dreamed of being a dancer. In my final year of study in the Contemporary Arts Program at Simon Fraser University, my body began to betray me. I had trained hard for four years, had performed, and had my choreography shown professionally even before I graduated from the program. I lived and breathed dance, it was in every fibre of who I was . . . or who I thought I was.

After graduating on crutches and feeling as though my dreams were shattered or certainly postponed, my entire life began to take a different route. A continual stream of injuries and health issues continued for over a decade, opening the doors (or rather shoving me through them) to my deep pursuit of Ayurveda.

Dance is something that I have always wanted to return to, but after living with Post-Viral Fatigue Syndrome for seven years I was scared to over exert myself, knowing how detrimental it could be.

Today I went to a Five Rhythms Dance class for the first time ever. The music came on and we were guided to use the breath to move the various parts of our body. It was like my body was waking up from a long sleep and returning to life. I allowed.

I allowed myself to move and be moved in any way I needed to without caring how I looked. All I cared was about how good it felt to move my body through space, to music, with sweat on my back and my hair flinging around my face. Energy began to flood through me and I welcomed it in and let it know it was safe to stay awhile. My body spiralled, flung, jumped; I felt like screaming out, "I AM HOME!"

What I realized this morning was that through all of my "spiritual" pursuits and austerities I feel most connected to myself and to life when I am dancing.

Dance is my Yoga.

Dance is my meditation.

Dance is my worship.

Dance is my healer.

Dance is my spirit, expressing purely and honestly without apology, excuse or shame.

For years I thought God was punishing me because my body wasn't doing what I wanted it to do, and wouldn't allow me to dance. During this incubation period of not dancing, I now realize that I no longer need to define myself as a dancer but I prefer to allow myself to be danced. That is the freedom.

> Dance, when you're broken open
> Dance, if you've torn the bandage off
> Dance in the middle of the fighting
> Dance in your blood
> Dance when you're perfectly free.
> ~ Rumi

Chapter 27

Fall Routines

Seasonal and Daily Practices for Fall

Routines are designed by Nature to stabilize, nurture, and nourish us.

How exhilarating it is when Summer turns to Fall. The air is crisp and fresh. Colours are earthy, deep, rich, and warm. The body is transitioning from saucy Summer sensuality to brisk Fall action and movement.

Swift, mobile, and light.

The body LOVES and responds to routine with glowing health. A daily practice for Fall brings the much needed stability, which is most important for thriving within the mutable nature of this season.

For some Fall can be an exhilarating transition, and for others it can be a whirlwind that can lift you spinning into mid air (or at least it can feel like that). There is a lot of activity and movement, as well as a dryness and a cool lightness in the air.

The most challenging thing to do at this time of year may be to implement routine and to stay present with the changing season.

Begin simply, as always. Choose, and set in place, your routines for the day. These are your anchors, which bring you to a balanced and grounded place. There is a temptation to do everything all at once. Keep it simple. Commit to staying with the practices that work best for you. Each day we have the opportunity to create a sustainable routine that will benefit and reward us in the long term with the good health we need to accomplish our life goals and thrive.

We cannot fake good health, but we do get to choose great health. One day at a time.

1. Start by waking a little later than in the Summer by about half an hour, around the same time each morning, setting your alarm to get you in the habit, and then eventually waking naturally with your internal clock. As the mornings are darker in the Fall, we shift into waking between 6:30 and 7:30 a.m. Some days you may just need more sleep in the morning. Most importantly, aim for allowing yourself enough time to do your morning practices while still getting ready for your day in a graceful way without rushing. Resist the temptation to multi-task. Bring mindful awareness to each practice.

2. Morning cleansing rituals: scrape tongue, brush teeth, start your oil pulling practice by swishing one tbsp sesame oil around the teeth and gums.

3. Drink warm water with a squeeze of lemon to assist elimination and cleanse the colon.

4. Massage sesame oil gently into both nostrils using either a cotton bud or your baby finger to apply the oil. This will help to alleviate dry nostrils and keep bacteria at bay.

5. Beautiful Body and Happy "Mind-Fall" Practices:

    - Meditate. (Even five minutes is a good start).

    - Breathe. Follow your Fall *pranayama* practice.

    - Move. (Follow your Fall yoga practice, dance, walk, cycle, stretch). Mindful movement in the Fall will stabilize you and set you up for a calm and effective day. Be careful not to overdo it. Consistency is more important in this erratic season than extreme activity.

    - Self-massage with warm sesame oil will tonify and nourish the skin and keep it from drying out.

    - Anoint yourself with EOs for the Fall. Choose from nutmeg, cardamom, vetiver, sweet orange, neroli, cardamom basil, spikenard, chamomile, lemon, myrrh, eucalyptus, geranium, lavender, sandalwood (refer to Fall Aromatherapy for application).

6. Meals: Breakfast, lunch, and dinner taken at the same times each day will benefit the nervous system and assist good digestion. Warm nourishing meals are best in the Fall with a focus on sweet, sour, and salty tastes with extra oils such as sesame, avocado, and olive added to meals.

    Breakfast: Warm and nourishing, eaten by 9 a.m.
    Lunch: Main meal, easy to digest, and eaten around midday.
    Dinner: Light, warm, and nourishing, ideally eaten by 6 p.m.

Before bed, take some quiet time for at least an hour of distraction-free space. Meditate, journal, pray, chant. Choose an activity that integrates your day and brings a peaceful night sleep. Rest is a biggie for soothing and restoring the nervous system, as well as detoxifying and healing the body and mind. Relax and nurture yourself. Aim for bedtime by 10 p.m.

Instill routines that inspire and stabilize to keep you thriving in the Fall!

Chapter 28

Fall Food Practices

The Fall season is the perfect opportunity to make sure we are getting enough oils and good fats in our diet. These lubricate our joints, and bring warmth and peace to a disturbed/overactive mind and nervous system.

The word for fat or oil in Sanskrit is *sneha* (which also translates as love). We need internal and external oleation during this season to nourish, protect, and insulate us from the cold dry elements.

As the leaves twirl ceaselessly from the trees, we need to be grounded and calm to navigate the whirlwind that defines this season. Our food suggestions are meant to nourish and pacify the predominant elements of air and ether as these are vulnerable and most likely to go out of balance in the Fall and early Winter.

The concept of eating seasonally is designed by Nature in such a way that no matter what your personal constitution, these practices work for you. Moderation is the key; awareness is the doorway. As with any of our practices, it is not helpful to go supernova and over tax our system. This approach leads to burnout and is a sure way to be thrown out of balance. The simplicity of a Fall practice revolves around sustainable routines with your mealtimes incorporating warm, sweet, nourishing foods.

What happens to our body and mind in the Fall? Remembering the qualities of the season and those of the *vata dosha*, we may observe dryness, cold, excess movement, sensitive nervous system, confusion, possible insomnia, stiffness in the joints, scattered thoughts, dry digestion, and anxiety. By refining our habits through these seasonal food practices, we can avoid getting derailed.

Feeding the mind first will alleviate stress, and avoid "*vata* derangement." By stocking up your spice and herb apothecary, you can be sure to have on hand just the right ingredients to keep you calm and present with your diet. Aromatic spices and herbs address the mind first through aroma nutrition, and once ingested, they work magically on the digestive system—enhancing appetite, digestion, and nutrient assimilation.

Balancing the six tastes is key in each season. We just need look around to gain clues to our ideal diet. Bright orange sweet pumpkins, squash, root vegetables, sweet pears, apples, persimmons, and plums are prominent at the Farmers' Markets and on grocery shelves. In the Fall, we balance our bodies with the predominant sweet, sour, and salty tastes as these bring moisture, warmth, and a strong digestive fire.

The sweet taste also builds and strengthens bones and bodily tissues, nourishes *ojas* (our life sap), and enhances the complexion. Without the sweet taste, we are grumpy, feel deprived, and cannot sustain grounded, calm emotions. We also need to include enough of the bitter, pungent, and astringent tastes so we do not accumulate sticky toxins in the body that will be harder to eliminate.

At this dry, cold time of year, we need more healthy, nourishing fats in our diet. Include sweet, heavy root veggies, and oily, heavy nut butters such as almond or cashew butter. We need warm, nutritive, calming foods such as hot soups, stews, mineral broths, stewed fruits, and nourishing cooked whole grains such as oats, wheat, rice, tapioca, wild fish, organic chicken, sweet roasted root vegetables, and steamed greens with healthy rich oil dressings. These are just a few of the food ideas for Fall. You get the idea—warm, nourishing, lubricating, sweet, calming, and soothing. Fall is not the time to deprive our bodies and souls of love!

All the herbs and spices listed below are beneficial to add to your meals. Along with a squeeze of lemon, these additions bring delicious flavour and ensure the benefits of all six tastes in balanced amounts.

Tip: Raw, cold foods like raw salads and raw vegetables, cold smoothies, and juices aggravate us in the cold season and hinder digestion setting up a cycle of imbalance. Avoid (or eat in moderation) drying foods such as crackers, popcorn, cold raw salads, and meals with no fats. Enjoy hearty snacks to appease afternoon cravings. A baked sweet potato around 3 p.m. with some ghee and spices is a wonderful way to get the serotonin levels registering in the brain—and much better than the fake-out energy boost of refined sugar highs.

Serotonin regulates our moods, grounds us, and keeps us cheerful. It is also essential for controlling the appetite and preventing a pattern of over-eating. We know when we are satisfied and so does the body. Empty nutrition from white refined sugar, refined flours, and sweets leech minerals from the bones and only offer us a quick fix energy boost, which leads to a cycle of addiction and cravings.

In Fall, as with almost any other time of the year, good carbohydrates are necessary to sustain us and keep our bodies in balance. That's the healthy, sweet taste we are talking about in an Ayurvedic lifestyle.

Tonic: Enjoy a mineral-rich, sweet, and salty broth for daily sipping to fortify you against the chilly, dry days. Simmer in a big pot for at least an hour: root veggies, peels, seeds from fall squash, sweet potato, beets, and yams, and add some kombu or other sea veggie, too. Strain the broth and add salt. Put your tonic in a flask and enjoy throughout the day.

Treat: Fall Bliss Balls. You may need a sweet and nourishing snack in the afternoon. These easy-to-make treats will boost your energy and ward off sugar cravings.

1 cup dates
3 tbsp tahini (sesame paste)
1/4 tsp ground nutmeg
1/2 tsp ground cinnamon
Sesame seeds for rolling

1. Soak dates 15 minutes in a bowl of boiled water until soft.

2. Remove date pits if not already pitted. Strain and remove from water. Mash well.

3. Stir in the tahini, mixing well. Mix in nutmeg and cinnamon.

4. Roll into small balls, and plop into sesame seeds to coat.

Fall Food Guide

Herb and Spice Magic for the Fall

Ajwan	Allspice	Anise	Asafoetida	Basil
*Black Pepper	Caraway	Cardamom	Cinnamon	*Cloves
Coriander	Cumin	Dill	Fennel	Fenugreek
Garlic	Ginger (fresh)	Mace	Nutmeg	Orange Peel
Oregano	Paprika	Parsley	Poppy Seeds	Rosemary
Saffron	Sage	Savory	Star Anise	Tamarind
Tarragon	Thyme	Turmeric		

*In moderation

Fall Legumes

Aduki Beans	Chickpeas	Lentils	Mung Beans	Tofu

Fall Grains

Amaranth	Barley	Oats	Pasta (wheat, rice)	Rice (all types)
*Quinoa	Spelt	Tapioca	Wheat Berries	Wheat

*In moderation

Fall Fruits

Apples (stewed/cooked)		Apricots	Avocado	Dates
Berries (cooked/fresh)		Figs	Grapefruit	Grapes
Lemons		Limes	Oranges	Plums	Pears
Raisins		Rhubarb		

Fall Veggies (mostly cooked)

Beets	Bell Pepper	*Brussel Sprouts	Carrots	Cauliflower
Fennel	Green Beans	Okra	Olives	Onions
Parsnip	Potato	Pumpkin	Rutabaga	Sea Veggies
Squash (All Seasonal Squash)		Salad Greens: Kale, Chard, Mustard Greens Etc. (Cooked/Steamed)		
Sweet Potato	Yams	Zucchini		

*In moderation

Fall Dairy

Butter	Cows Milk	Cream	Ghee	Goats Cheese
Goats Milk	Yoghurt			

Fall Fish and Meat

Beef	Bison	Chicken (with skin)	Duck	
Fish (freshwater)	Salmon	Sardines	Shellfish	
Tuna	Turkey (mostly dark meat)			

Fall Nuts* Seeds and Condiments

Almonds (soaked and peeled)	Brazil Nuts	Cashews	Coconut
Flax Seed	Hazelnuts	Hemp Seed	Macadamia	Pumpkin Seeds
Pine Nuts	Sesame Seeds	Sunflower Seeds		

*Soaking your nuts in water overnight and then peeling off the skin allows for better digestion. Nuts and seeds naturally contain enzyme inhibitors, which are indigestible and therefore create toxins in the system. Only soak the amount you are going to eat that day to avoid mold and fermentation.

Fall Oils

Almond	Avocado	Canola	Ghee	
Olive	Sesame	Sunflower		

Fall Sweeteners

Brown Rice Syrup	Brown Sugar (Unrefined)	Cane Sugar (Raw, Unprocessed)	Dates	
Fruit Juice Concentrates	Honey (Raw Is Best)	Molasses	Maple Syrup	

Fall Teas

Basil (Tulsi/Holy Basil)	Cardamom	Chai	Cinnamon
Ginger	Licorice	Orange Peel	Sage
*CCF (Classic Ayurvedic tea of cumin, coriander and fennel)			

*To make CCF tea take 1 tsp each of fennel seed, cumin seed, and coriander seed. Add along with 4 cups water to a small pot and bring to boil. When mixture has reached a boil, turn down to simmer for 10-15 minutes. Strain and drink. This tea is cleansing, aids the digestive system and supports the absorption of nutrients in the body while bringing the body into a state of acid/alkaline (pH) balance. A great tea to reset the body after any over-indulgences.

Fall Meal Ideas and Recipes

Breakfast: Sweet grains are a good warming breakfast. Add spices, seeds, nuts, and dried fruits from your Fall Food Guide for a satisfying meal to start your day off right. Add 1 tsp of ghee.

- Savory breakfasts such as rice with miso or mineral broth can be a good first meal of the day.

- Experiment with other seasonal grains, or try poached/boiled eggs with avocado on wheat toast with ghee.

- Try breakfast compote with stewed fruits, ghee, and tahini on top.

Lunch: This should be your main meal of the day as digestion is at its prime between noon and 2 p.m.

- Remember to include all six tastes for a balanced and satisfying meal.

- Soups, stews, and warm hearty lunches will give you the strength and support you need.

- Sweet root veggies with ghee, steamed greens with oil dressings, grains, and mung bean soups or small portions of animal foods make up a good lunch.

- Experiment with a variety of foods from the Fall Food Guide.

Dinner: This can be a lighter meal taken at least three hours before bedtime.

- Enjoy a variety of spices and condiments with your meal to include all six tastes.

- Soups, grains, small portions of animal foods, and a rotating variety of veggies is best.

- Simplicity is key for your daily evening meal. Focus on the sweet, sour, and salty tastes.

- Eat slowly and enjoy every bite. Offer gratitude before each meal.

Butternut Harvest Moon Soup

Serves 4

3lb large butternut squash
1 large yam

1 medium onion
2 tbsp ghee or sesame oil
8 cups water or veggie broth
2 tbsp fresh grated ginger
2 tbsp finely grated orange rind
1 tsp ground fennel seeds
1 tsp ground coriander
1 tsp sea salt
1 tsp lemon juice
Pumpkin seeds and fresh sage for garnish

1. Cut butternut squash in half and put face down on foil in roasting dish.
2. Bake in oven at 375º F for half an hour. When squash is soft, remove skin and seeds and set aside.
3. Sauté one medium diced onion with 2 tbsp ghee or sesame oil in a medium pot for 2 minutes until onion partly browns.
4. Add 8 cups water or veggie broth and bring to boil with lid on.
5. Peel and dice yam and add to pot lowering heat and cooking for 5 minutes.
6. Add in the roasted squash.
7. Add fresh grated ginger, finely grated orange rind, ground fennel seeds, ground coriander, and stir in.
8. Blend with a hand-held blender or regular blender and purée to a creamy consistency. Thin soup out with more water if needed.
9. Add sea salt and lemon juice and stir.
10. Garnish with finely chopped fresh sage and pumpkin seeds. Enjoy!

This soup is very sweet, warming, and wonderful for the chillier Fall season.

A Nutritive Fall *Masala*

Spices! A great way to get all six tastes in each meal and to experience amazingly delicious and aromatic food is to add a lively balanced *masala* (spice blend). Doing this satisfies all the senses and signals a message of satisfaction to the brain, making it less likely to over-eat. We need warming, sweet, and grounding spices such as the ones listed in the Fall Food Guide. Sesame seeds anchor the blend and add power-packed nutrients as well.

1 cup sesame seeds
1 tsp coriander seeds
1 tsp cumin seed
1 tsp fennel seeds
1/4 tsp cardamom seeds, already removed from pods
1/2 tsp ground cinnamon

1/8 tsp salt

1. On medium heat in a cast iron skillet or heavy frying pan, lightly toast the sesame seeds until they "crackle and pop" and turn a light golden brown.
2. With a mortar and pestle or a blender, gently crack the seeds being careful not to pulverize them. They are best crunchy, so over-blending will turn them into sesame paste.
3. Pour into a bowl.
4. Toast together the cumin, coriander, fennel, and cardamom seeds being careful not to burn them. They can go from raw to burned quickly. You will notice their exquisite scent is released when they are ready. Once again in your mortar and pestle or blender, grind the seeds until they are almost powdered but still slightly crunchy.
5. Add to sesame seeds. Add cinnamon and salt.
6. Meld spice blend together.

Sweet, warm, salty, and heavenly fragrant! Sprinkle lavishly on rice, veggies, soups, salads etc.

Tridoshic Fall *Kichari*

Serves 3-4

One of the best ways to give your over taxed digestive system a break is to eat *kichari*, an Ayurvedic superfood. *Kichari* is a *tridoshic* (good for all *dosha* types) food that can be adjusted according to the season or for your individual constitution.

The basic ingredients in this one pot meal are white basmati rice and split mung beans. These ingredients form a complete protein and are very easily digested. Added to the pot are spices to help kindle your digestive fire, as well as yummy veggies for good nourishment.

This powerful dish is the staple for an Ayurvedic cleanse diet, but can also be used anytime you feel your digestion is out of whack. Eating *kichari* is like pressing the reset button and allows your digestion to return to a state of proper functioning and ease.

6 cups water, may add more water for a more soupy *kichari*
2 tbsp ghee—see ghee recipe in Summer Recipe section
Half a medium onion, finely diced
1 inch fresh peeled ginger, finely diced
1 cup split mung dal
1 cup white basmati rice
About 2 cups mixed veggies of your choice—seasonal root veggies, squash, and greens
1 tsp asafoetida
1 tsp cumin seeds

1 tsp coriander seeds
1 tsp fennel seeds
1 tsp sea salt or rock salt

Tip: Soak beans and rice overnight in cold water for shorter cooking time and easier digestion.

1. Wash beans and rice until rinse water is clear. Discard water and set rice and beans aside.
2. In a heavy-bottomed pan, heat the ghee on medium and add the onions to sauté until sweet and tender.
3. Add ginger, cumin, fennel, asafoetida, and coriander seeds and sauté for two or so more minutes.
4. Add rice and beans and sauté for a few more minutes.
5. Add the water, cover and bring to a boil. Once boiling, stir, lower heat and simmer on low with the lid on for about 20 minutes.
6. While *kichari* is cooking, wash and chop the veggies/greens.
7. Add to the mixture, stir in and cover.
8. Allow to steam for about 8-10 minutes. Add salt and mix in. If you are using veggies that take longer to cook than greens—squash or yams for example—add to mixture five minutes before the greens and other veggies.

Garnish: A squeeze of lemon or lime, fresh cilantro or parsley, a small dollop of extra ghee, and toasted sesame seeds or toasted sunflower seeds. You can also use the Spicy Fall *Masala* recipe as a delicious condiment, sprinkling lavishly over your *kichari*.

This is just one suggested recipe for *kichari*. Feel free to adjust veggies and spices to suit your tastes. Get creative with it. Here's to simple eating and your health!

Fall Beddy-Bye Tonic for Good Sleep

To be taken half an hour before bed. Grate 1/8 tsp of nutmeg into 1/2 cup of warm milk or almond milk. Nutmeg is like a natural tranquilizer. Enjoy this tonic as it soothes the mind and encourages a restful night's sleep. Add a small amount of honey to sweeten if desired.

Chapter 29

Fall Self-Care

How does the Fall Season make you feel? Take a minute to contemplate this question. Is it the same every year? Do you notice more movement, distracted thinking, dry skin, and chilly extremities?

It is quite easy in Fall for any of us to sometimes feel like a crazed person trying to hang on to our hats for most of this season. Grounding our selves takes a ton of effort and mindfulness. Even though we know it is time to start winding down and quieting the din inside our heads, we are propelled to fly through the season in a dizzy spell of juggling, running, and doing.

A simplified and organized routine at this time of year empowers us to follow through with our daily self-care practices. This makes us feel calmer, more vibrant, and present.

The Fall season is all about movement and activity, so how do we then do less, stay still, and be quiet?

Take a moment to reflect upon this simple wisdom written by Henry David Thoreau, which tells us that staying calm whilst you are busy is not really about doing less, it is more about what you choose to do and how you choose to do it.

"It is not enough to be busy. So are the ants. The question is—what are we busy about?"

Mindfulness.

When done with mindfulness, all and any practices you take on for the Fall season—in fact, for all seasons of your life—transform the doing into being. There is the perfect Sanskrit word for the mindful daily practice: *sadhana*. This is a word that describes doing with being; the full presence, focus, and love poured into any and every task and activity you undertake.

These are the wholesome everyday practices observed in accordance with the rhythms and cycles of Nature offered with an attitude of love and devotion. Mother Maya defines *sadhana* in her book Women's Power to Heal through Inner Medicine as ". . . awareful practices that evoke our Inner Medicine healing potential and keep our inner rhythms in alignment with Mother Consciousness. This is the indestructible maternal energy imbued in each and every person, the central support that upholds the whole universe."

In short, mindful practices aligned with the cycles of Nature are what bring balance and a state of grace, joy, and symbiosis to your life. They accumulate and they count for the long-term. Mindful practices are comforting, unifying, and, above all else, harmonizing.

Your self-care for the Fall season is about warmth, sweetness, comfort, nourishment, and grounding. There is nothing more delectable for the body, mind, and soul than a warm, evening bath with salts and aromatic oils, nothing more nourishing then a flask of mineral broth sipped during the day to fortify against wind and overwhelm. Nothing is more grounding than the wafting of an earthy, aromatic oil reaching your nose, and then your brain, and then your heart and soul.

Choose two or three of these soul-care suggestions that resonate with you and establish them consistently in your daily routine.

Glowing Fall Face Cleanse

Face the world with a glow! Every day you see yourself in the mirror, your inner light shines through to reflect on the outside what is happening internally. Homemade face cleansers add a shine and feed your skin so you can feel confident you are using all natural ingredients in accordance with Nature, while honouring yourself and the environment.

Make enough for a week or two supply of this yummy cleanser for a fresh and moisture-rich skin. Use in the morning to cleanse your skin.

Dry ingredients

1 cup finely ground wheat germ flakes (or substitute oats if wheat allergies are a concern)
1/2 cup unhulled, finely ground sesame seeds
1 cup dried milk powder
1 tbsp ground dried orange peel

Blend together, store in an airtight glass jar in a cool dry place or in the refrigerator.

Wet ingredients

Sesame seed oil (cold pressed, untoasted)
Water or orange blossom water

Keep separate and add to dry mix to make into a creamy paste for each cleansing application.

For your daily morning face cleansing ritual, take 1 tbsp of the dry mixture and add to 1/2 tsp sesame oil and enough water or orange blossom water to mix into a creamy thick paste. With upward sweeping and circular strokes massage over entire neck and face. Add more liquid if necessary to get a smooth application. Without scrubbing, gently massage your face. Wash off with warm water, and gently pat skin dry with a clean towel.

Nutritious Fall Face Moisturizer

Make enough for a week or two supply of this rich moisturizer for soft, smooth, and warm skin. Use in the morning to moisturize and nourish your skin.

Mix together and store in an airtight glass bottle:

1 cup unrefined cold-pressed sesame oil
12 drops neroli or sweet orange EO
12 drops geranium EO
5 drops lemon EO

1 bottle orange blossom water to have on hand. Do not mix into oil blend.

Each morning after cleansing, take 1/2 tsp of oil blend and mix with 1 tsp orange blossom water, or regular filtered water, and massage into face.

Sweet Sleep Salt Soak

Aaaaah, a warm, aromatic bath at the end of a cold Fall day! Add some love to your bathwater and embrace yourself with a fragrant soak before heading to bed for a restful sleep to quiet and relax the active *vata* mind. Enjoy at least twice a week.

Make enough for a week supply—about 4 baths:

1 cup Epsom salts
1 cup sea salt
1/4 cup sesame oil
1/4 cup almond oil
20 drops geranium EO
5 drops clary sage EO
5 drops sweet orange EO

Mix together, and store in airtight glass jar. Use 1/2 cup aromatic oil salt soak in each bath.

Sweet Dreams!

Fall Aromatherapy. How Sweet It Is.

Every season brings an opportunity to make friends with the healing plant essences. In the Fall, we use essential oils to warm and soothe the frenetic, dry, cold qualities of the time of year that can deplete our body and make us feel anxious, chaotic, and out of balance.

Aromatherapy in the Fall stabilizes the mind and brings calm to the emotions, providing restoration and peace. It is a deeply effective way to bring focus and stability to your system so that you can enjoy the benefits and beauty of the season.

Slowly build your aromatherapy apothecary for each season, and you will always have a remedy on hand. The oils are versatile and can be blended in a multitude of ways.

Suggested Essential Oil List for Fall
(Sweet, calming, grounding, regulating, warming, peaceful)

Stock your bathroom apothecary with at least three or four of these fragrant friends: ginger, spikenard, clary sage, bergamot, sweet orange, vetiver, lavender, rose, sandalwood, rosewood, geranium, lemon, cardamom, jasmine, and/or neroli.

How to include aromatherapy in your daily Fall practice:

Make a pure essential oil blend using two or three different oils. Store in a dark glass airtight bottle. You can also keep four or five different essential oils in your bathroom cabinet and blend as needed or use individually as preferred.

1. Massage oil: By adding an essential oil blend to a carrier oil, you can have a customized massage blend on hand to use as needed. Two lovely massage carrier oils are sesame or almond oil (or an equal mix of the two). You can also use half sunflower and half sesame for a lighter oil. A ratio of between 48-90 drops of pure essential oil to 4 oz carrier oil is the standard range depending on how potent you want your blend. Keep your blend simple when starting out, using only 3 or 4 essential oils. Play and experiment as you discover the best scents for you.

2. Bath oil: The best way to use essential oils in the bath is to mix them with salts or an emulsifier such as milk or your chosen carrier oil. You can also add your custom massage blend directly into the bath. Two to three tablespoons would make for a luxurious bath and allow the oils to be absorbed deeply into the skin.

A good ratio is 10-20 drops essential oil mixed with 1/2 cup of salts or emulsifier.

Aromatic baths in the Fall are excellent for helping bring both harmony and quiet to the central nervous system and the mind.

3. Direct Palm Inhalation: Apply 1-2 drops of essential oil directly to the palms, rub together gently and inhale deeply. This is an excellent method to gain quick and easy exposure to the essential oils.

4. Facial steam: Place 1-3 drops in a bowl of steaming hot water, cover head with a towel, steam face. Excellent for alleviating stress and anxiety. Geranium, lavender, and neroli or sweet orange are particularly good at this time of year.

G & M's Fall Journals

G

October 16th

My kitchen is my apothecary of delights. It is my haven and my playground. I revel in the sensuality that comes from working with the aromatic herbs and spices. Every spice is like a friend, unique in personality, character and fragrance. When you put them all together in different combinations they transform the experience, just as a gathering of friends would. Each bringing a flavor unlike any other. The nutmeg dense and sweet, intoxicating and serious. The cardamom sensual and aromatic, romantic and inviting. The coriander sensible, friendly and accessible. The ginger feisty and full of stories to tell.

The seeds and spices are so sure—sure of who they are and what they contribute. They know where they come from and what is their purpose. They do not shy away from authentically offering themselves as they are. They understand that their contribution is transformative.

We are much like them, only we seem to forget. That is why I love to party with them. Only one small whiff and I am filled with remembrance.

M

October 24th

Throughout my "spiritual" quest, there were times I became so disillusioned that I believed that there was a right way to do life, a right way to reach enlightenment and, essentially, be safe. I gave my power over to men claiming to be enlightened and was told if I got my ego out of the way and let them take advantage of me they would grant me enlightenment. Nothing could be further from the truth. It is heartbreaking to think that at times I was so naïve, or perhaps so deeply longing to reconnect to something that has always been within me.

I had forgotten that I am the light.

I see this everywhere I go—the disconnection that so many people have with life. We have forgotten that, here, we are Spirit, in this beautiful human form, and that no one can take away our light or give us anything because Divinity is built in, it's not an add on. No one is any more spiritual than anyone else. In fact, I think that word, "spiritual," is quite ridiculous as it automatically sets up a distinction between things that are not spiritual. This is the trap. This was my blind spot.

I needed to let go of the striving to be more, to be better, perfect, in hopes that the Divine would then recognize how bloody hard I had tried to be good. Spirit doesn't want us to be good, Spirit wants us to be ourselves and express the magnificence that we are. We came here whole, uniquely profound, and now we must be THAT.

It's easier than we think.

Stop all the craziness, all the incessant lies we tell ourselves that we're not good enough, smart enough, rich enough. It's time to open our eyes and wake up to the richness and beauty within. When we're able to tap into this ever flowing experience, we see and feel the beauty all around us. We abide in the firm knowing that everything is going exactly according to plan in the universe.

Chapter 30

Fall Yoga, *Pranayama*, and Meditation Practices

Yoga to Keep Your Feet On the Ground

Use your Fall yoga flow to bring balance to your over-stimulated nervous system, overwhelmed mind, and stressed out body. You will reap great benefits with a consistent daily practice as you develop physical strength and mental equanimity.

To reduce *vata* at this time of year, practice your yoga in a calm, slow, and steady way. Let go of your inner flailing orangutan that may resist stillness and pause. Imagine yourself as a 100 year-old Chinese Tai Chi Master moving with agility, grace, and ease.

> **Fall Flow Tips**
>
> ~ Practice at the same time every day to generate routine.
> ~ Be consistent.
> ~ Best time to practice: Sunrise to 10a.m., 2 to 6p.m.
> ~ Anytime is better then none at all.
> ~ Manage your energy with slow, calm, and steady breathing in and out through your nose.

Yoga Time

This practice is short and succinct and can be done in approximately 20 minutes so that you can fit it into your busy day. Some yoga is better than no yoga, and it is the consistent practice that will offer you the changes and transformation you're looking for.

1. Low Back Lovin'
(2 min.)
Begin by lying on your back. Bend your knees and draw them in towards your chest. Clasp your hands around your knees or shins. Rock slowly and gently from side to side, massaging your lower back. Keep the knees together and circle them in one direction and then the other as you continue to relax your lower back area.

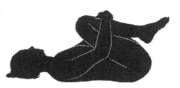

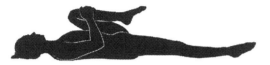

2. Wind releasing...yes, that's right (*Pawanmuktasana*: Wind Releasing)
(1 min.)
Keep your right leg bent into your chest and extend your left leg straight out on the floor. Hands remain clasped around the knee or shin of the right leg. Breathe slowly and deeply here (3-5 breaths) as the ascending colon is massaged, improving digestion and elimination. Exhale, release the right leg straight out on the floor. Inhale—draw the left leg towards the chest, massaging the descending colon (3-5 breaths).
Exhale—release the left leg to the ground.

3. Twist it Sista' (*Jathara Parivartasana*: Spinal Twist)
(2 min.)
Stay lying on your back with your knees bent and together with your feet flat on the floor. Interlace your fingers together and clasp your hands behind your head, cupping the back of your head in your hands. Inhale. As you exhale take the bent knees over to the floor on the right side, creating a beautiful twist through your spine. If it's comfortable, turn your head to look in the opposite direction from the bent knees. Breathe here for 3-5 breaths. Inhale to bring your knees back to the starting position. Exhale—repeat on the second side.

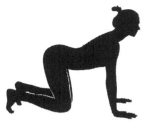
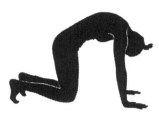

4. The Cat's Meow (*Marjariasana*: Cat Stretch)
(1 min.)
Come up onto your hands and knees. Place your shoulders directly above your wrists and hips above your knees. Spread your finger bones open like fans and press the entire surface of your hands into the floor. Inhale—begin by tipping your tailbone towards the sky and dipping your abdomen towards the earth. Continue to sequence through the spine until your chest and gaze are also looking upwards. Exhale—draw your tailbone down to point towards the ground as you lift your navel up towards the ceiling, dropping the head in to the chest. Repeat 5X.

5. Child's Pose…Aaaaawh (*Balasana*: Pose of the Child)
(1 min.)
Press your buttocks back to sit on your heels, resting your forehead on the ground (if your buttocks do not rest on your heels, place a pillow or folded blanket in between them so that you can relax). Bring your arms by your sides, palms upwards with the elbows slightly bent. Breathe slowly and deeply into the belly 5-10X.

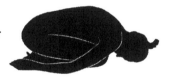

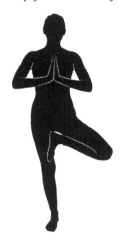

6. Tree balance…Insert sense of humour here (*Vriksasana*: Tree)
(1 min.)
Stand with your weight equally on both feet. Begin to shift your body weight towards the right foot. Place the ball of the left foot to the right ankle or on the side of the right calf or inner thigh (not beside the right knee). Keep your pelvis square to the front of the room. Hands come together in front of your heart or above your head. Breathe comfortably here as you balance on one foot. Smile. Stay as long as you can. Repeat on the second side.

7. Triangle (*Trikonasana*: Triangle)
(2 min.)

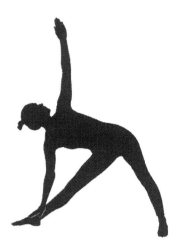

Start by standing with both feet together. Take the left leg back approximately 3-4 feet and place the left foot on a forward angle of about 45 degrees. Inhale—raise both arms up to shoulder height. Exhale—shift the weight of your pelvis towards the left as you reach to the side with the torso and right arm (keeping both sides of the torso long and even). Place the right hand on the right leg without collapsing your body weight into it. Look up towards the left hand (if this is uncomfortable for your neck, look down to the floor). Breathe here for 5 full breaths. Inhale to press into your feet, engage your abdominal muscles and return upright. Exhale—lower your hands to your hips. Inhale step the left foot forward beside the right foot.

Repeat on the second side.

8. Divine Restoration (*Viparita Karani* Variation: Legs up the wall)
(3-5 min.)

Sit sideways with your right hip against the wall. Use the support of your hands to gently roll yourself onto your back with your legs up against the wall. Your sitting bones should touch the wall here. Relax your entire upper body as your legs stay extended up the wall in alignment with your hips. Close your eyes. Relax the face, jaw, shoulders, belly, and legs. Breathe into your abdomen and lower back area.

To come out of this restorative posture, bend your knees and push your feet into the wall to slide back away from it. Turn onto one side and use your arms to slowly push yourself upright.

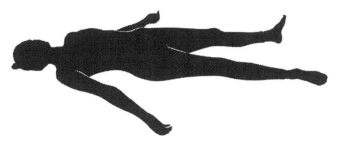

13. Icing on the Cake (*Savasana*—Corpse Pose)
(10 min.)
Savasana is the most important yoga posture, especially to reduce elevated vata. It helps to relax and balance the whole nervous system and allows time to integrate all of the benefits from your yoga practice into your mind and body.

Lay down on your back with your head and spine straight, legs apart, letting the feet flop out to the sides. Arms are away from the sides of the body slightly, and the palms face upward. (Use a bolster under the knees if your lower back is sore, and cover up with a blanket to stay warm if needed.) Close your eyes.

Let your entire body relax. Begin at your toes and relax your feet. Move your awareness up through the body all the way to the head, consciously letting go of any stress or tension along the way. The breath is completely natural. Surrender into the stillness and silence of this posture.

Once you have completed the practice, start to wiggle your fingers and toes. Stretch your body in any way that feels great. Roll to one side and use your hands to push you to an upright position.

The Attitude of Gratitude: Don't Leave Home Without It

- Notice how you are feeling.

- How has this simple yoga practice transformed your body and mind?

- Before jumping up and carrying on with your day, take a moment to acknowledge your efforts and commitment to your practice.

- Bring your hands together in front of your heart. Close your eyes. Appreciate whatever it is that brings you love and joy in your life.

- Honour and thank yourself for showing up and doing your yoga today.

Balance Your Brain Just By Breathing

We need only look as far as our breathing patterns to understand the state of our mind, and where we hold tension in the body. Our breath is intrinsically connected to our nervous system; therefore, conscious breathing is one of the most powerful ways to transform stress, anxiety, and overwhelm into peace, calm, and clarity. A daily *pranayama*, or conscious breathing practice, is the arsenal you need to blow your negative thinking habits to smithereens (with loving kindness, of course).

The technique of *nadi shodhana*, or alternate nostril breathing as it is often called, is a purifying breath. In Sanskrit, *nadi* means channel or flow of energy, and *shodhana* means purification. This simple yet powerful technique balances the two hemispheres of the brain, nourishes the body with extra oxygen, and releases carbon dioxide and toxins from the system. Stress and anxiety are decreased through the clearing of *pranic* blockages that lead to dis-ease. When our *prana*, our vital energy is balanced we have great focus, clarity, tranquility, and ease.

This is a wonderful practice to do before bed to help with sleep, or at any time that you feel off centre. The impact that *nadi shodhana* has on the nervous system feels instant and palpable and powerfully transforms instability to stability and agitation to ease.

The How-To of Alternate Nostril Breathing (*Nadi Shodhana*)

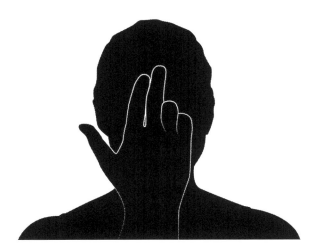

1. Sit in a chair in a comfortable position or cross-legged on the floor; wherever you can have an elongated spine.

2. Establish a slow, calm, and steady breathing pattern in and out of your nostrils.

3. Bring your right hand into *Nasagra Mudra*. That is, rest the index and middle fingers of your right hand gently at your eyebrow centre. The thumb is in front of the right nostril and the ring finger above the left. The thumb and ring fingers control the flow of breath in the nostrils by alternately closing off one nostril at a time.

4. Close off your right nostril with your thumb and inhale through the left nostril. Simultaneously count mentally, "One, two, three, four, five . . ." until the inhalation ends comfortably.

5. Close the left nostril with your ring finger and exhale out through the right nostril to the same count, "One, two, three, four, five . . ." until the exhalation ends comfortably (your inhalation and exhalation should have the same count).

6. Now, inhale through the right nostril, again with the same count. At the top of the breath, close the right nostril by pressing the thumb to close it and exhale out through the left nostril. This is one full round. Practice nine more rounds.

Practice Tips

- Never force or strain with your breathing practice, it should always feel natural and comfortable.

- After practicing *nadi shodhana* for a couple of weeks, you may wish to increase the length of your inhalation and exhalation by one count.

- Over time, as your lung capacity expands and nervous system strengthens, you can increase the count bit by bit.

So-Ham Meditation: Your Fall Lifeline

M

Sitting still and doing nothing gets a bad rap in our culture. It is equated to laziness and lack of productivity. I was indoctrinated into the world of goal-oriented accomplishments at a young age as my Mother always had to-do lists for us on days off school; cleaning and "pulling our weight" around the house was insisted upon.

When I wasn't cleaning the house, I was out doing something. Be it dance class, swimming lessons, field hockey practice or practicing the saxophone . . . you name it and I was probably doing it. There is nothing inherently wrong with doing—except if we are constantly just getting things done then we are incapable of just being. Just being is a skill to be mastered.

Being is the black belt of spiritual practice.

My very first visit to see an Ayurvedic doctor was a fairly anti-climactic event. I had just been through some serious health problems that he seemed to overlook. He did, however, leave me with a golden nugget of wisdom that to this day is priceless (and likely gets to the root cause of my health concerns).

He said to me, "You need to learn to get your sense of self-worth not from what you do, but from who you are."

At the time I didn't pay much attention to this comment, however, over the years it has seeped down into my cells and sprung back up like a whisper, a hum, and a clear voice that has more wisdom in it than all of my years of doing.

In essence, I was burning myself out as I strove to do, achieve, and get somewhere other then where I was—thinking I would somehow be a better person and on a deeper, subconscious level, perhaps more lovable.

At the core of our human existence, we want to be loved, and not only do we want to be loved, we yearn to be accepted as we are, with all of our quirks, foibles, and idiosyncrasies. Yet, we put a lot of energy into being someone we are not, holding up appearances and putting on our mask each day as we politely say, "Thank you," and "Yes, please," and "Sorry."

Keeping that mask up can be exhausting.

Being still and sitting silently may be excruciatingly agonizing. You may even feel like you are going crazy as you become a witness to the myriad of thoughts flashing across the screen of the mind—twirling, spinning, and spiraling with chaotic enthusiasm. At other times, a deep sense of peace will well up from the depths of your self, washing you clean with loving grace.

The trick is not to have preference over either of these states. Equanimity.

Equanimity takes practice, and will require all of your might not to judge yourself for whatever state you may be in. The trap is the illusion of progress on your spiritual path. You do not become spiritual; *you are* spiritual no matter what your life looks like. You can become more conscious, but your spiritual bank account is full by the sheer fact that you are alive and here on this planet having a human experience.

So relax!

Do you ever find yourself feeling overwhelmed in the Fall season? Busy, running here, there, and everywhere, and always feeling a step behind? Worn down? Worn out?

In Nature, the Fall time is a period of retraction or moving inwards. Seldom do we balance our hectic schedules with stillness and nourishment. Meditation is known as the first medicine in Ayurveda and is the key to wholeness and knowing ourselves beyond the persona that we have groomed over our lifetime.

Take some time everyday to do this meditation practice. It is an ancient healing mantra meditation that can be used anytime, anywhere. The mantra *So Ham* (pronounced so-hum) holds a sound frequency that is healing. This mantra translates as, "I am that," allowing us to contemplate on the great mystery of being. This meditation is thousands of years old and has been used by many great sages and saints to focus the mind, balance the emotions, and induce a rewiring of the nervous system.

Start off by dedicating 5-10 minutes a day to this practice. Allow this time to lengthen as you naturally experience the benefits of meditation. Using an alarm to mark the amount of time you would like to meditate that day is useful so that you do not become distracted wondering how long you have been practicing.

The How-To of the *So Ham* Meditation

1. Find a comfortable place to sit with your spine straight (in a chair, with your back against a wall, or cross-legged).

2. Place your hands face down on your thighs (to ground your energy) or in *Gyan Mudra*—your index finger curled in to touch the root of the thumb, palms down.

3. Close your eyes. Scan through your entire body with your awareness. Notice any places you may be holding any tension and invite these places to relax (you can mentally say, "Relax," to the various body parts as you let go of any tension or tightness there).

4. Breathing in and out of the nostrils, begin to slow your breath down. Let the breath be long and steady without any strain whatsoever. Once you feel established in this rhythm, mentally repeat to yourself, "Soooooooooooooo," on the inhalation and, "Huuuuuuummmmmm," on your exhalation.

5. At the end of your practice, place your hands in *Pranam Mudra*—your palms touching in front of your heart, and take a moment to consciously connect with someone or something that you are grateful for.

Practice Tip

If a thought arises, notice it, acknowledge it, and then let it go. Return to the mantra and to the awareness of your breath flowing in and out of the nostrils.

Chapter 31

Fall Ceremony and Ritual

G

There is something about this time of year that makes me notice colour more intensely. First, there is a luscious display of the early Fall—the harvest. The changing of the leaves is a palette of delight for visual feasting.

As I go on my daily morning walks, I stop and observe the mountains and the trees. Over the period of three months as I watch the transformation, I feel deeply connected with the concept of change and the beauty that exists if we just take time to notice it and are present with what is.

Towards the late Fall, the lake ices up, seemingly prematurely. The ducks skate-land on the lake on which, just a few days prior, they had been paddling through with ease. But they are still there, working with what is, staying together, and accommodating themselves according to Nature's changes. All these transformations in one season reveal the necessary fade and ephemeral decay of Fall.

This season witnessed and celebrated gives us pause.

I ponder how these outer changes reflect the inner changes. I turn this into a ceremony by burning some crushed dry leaves with aromatic agar wood, "the wish-fulfilling gem." This sacred wood is used for a ceremony which seals in your intentions once they have been sent out by prayer to the Cosmos.

The Fall season is a time for gratitude and giving, even if you feel you have very little to share.

These Autumn rituals are performed for giving thanks:

- To solidify our understanding of the close connections between our self, Nature, and the Cosmos.
- To express our reverence for Nature and the plenty of this season.
- To celebrate the beauty of all life and honour the changes.
- To see human life as an integral part of the Cosmos and the cycles of Nature.
- To strengthen our beliefs and intentions.
- To bring peace and stability in times of uncertainty.

The Cherokee First Nation's creation stories say that Fall was when the world was created and the great new moon in Fall (October) represented a celebration of the new year. This celebration gave birth to Thanksgiving—offering foods from the harvest, gathering together to share stories, sing and dance, and to offer gratitude to the Great Spirit. It was, and still very much is, a time to feast and offer thanks to the Creator for their blessings and for the cycles of the seasons to continue.

Our Thanksgiving here in North America is a beautiful time to reflect on the bounty of the harvest, the transitions in our own lives, and the thanks we can offer for all that we have. If you live in a place where this is not traditionally celebrated, you can create your own ritual of Thanksgiving during the Fall season.

Fall Ceremony Themes: Change, Harvest, Bounty, Gratitude

Create your Fall sacred space by incorporating some of the following objects: dried leaves, candles, branches, gourds, dried corn, and harvest symbols. Remove all of the Summer objects from your altar, and place a new Fall-coloured cloth or covering and other meaningful items to mark the season.

Write in your journal all that you are grateful for. Prepare a special meal using local seasonal foods. Gather leaves of all shapes, sizes, and colours, and press them by placing them in the middle of heavy books. In a week, they will be flat and dry and can be used for decorating, table displays, bookmarks, and your gratitude tree.

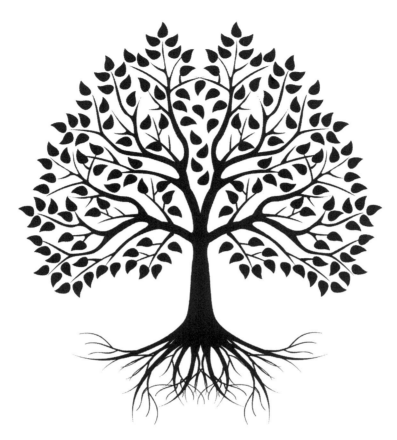

Photocopy and enlarge this tree symbol or create your own, and stick collected and dried pressed leaves from various trees to fill out your gratitude tree for your sacred space. Add to these leaves on your gratitude tree by cutting out your own leaf shapes from paper and writing on each one a different prayer or single word of gratitude.

When we give thanks and acknowledge all that we have, we receive abundance from the Universe and we release stuck patterns of negativity.

Create an intention for yourself and infuse that into everything you do for this season.

Set aside a special time for your ceremony or integrate it into your Thanksgiving day.

Allow yourself to celebrate and mark the season with your own personal ritual. This practice will awaken your senses and observations, and empower you to be present. These rituals can change as you transform, they will find a life of their own and align with you as an ally on your journey.

Madhuri Phillips and Glynnis Osher

As a sacred environment that is set up and energized with your intentions, your altar acts as the witness, holding the space for your ceremonies and rituals. Once you have set up your personal space for ritual, you may find that small miracles begin to happen. Awakenings may spark new ideas, feelings of joy, and motivation. If you have not already set up your altar space, now is a good time to do so.

Chapter 32

Fantastic 14-Day Fall Cleanse

Why a Fall Cleanse?

In Ayurveda, our body is looked upon as a sacred vessel taking us on a journey to the highest, most beloved beings we can be. We are guided to take care of this worthy vehicle with the utmost care, love, and respect. In this case, it is fitting that we treat our bodies well and maintain them as we would our most precious possessions.

A Fall cleanse is the perfect way to clear and tune our bodies, ridding us of accumulations and toxins that are obstacles to our irresistible life. Fall being the *vata* season, we need to focus on a cleansing practice that pacifies the air and ether elements. As the season is dry, windy, and cool, internal and external oleation serves to nourish, restore, and fortify the digestive and nervous system while boosting immunity.

A simple mono-diet of *kichari* benefits proper digestion, assimilation, and elimination to regain equilibrium of metabolic function. Sounds complicated? It is not.

This classic Ayurvedic cleansing food is also nourishing, satisfying, and simple; as well as being a complete protein combination of split mung beans and rice. Added spices aid in stoking the digestive fire and the ghee assists to dislodge and clear out sticky toxins (*ama*) away from the tissues to the digestive tract where they can be eliminated. Veggies complete this perfect detox dish providing fiber, color, and texture to the experience.

During the busy Fall season, this simple cleanse comes as a reprieve and will leave you feeling divinely restored.

Enjoy the Benefits:

- Improved digestion
- Clear skin
- More energy
- Better sleep
- Toned, flexible joints
- Healthy weight
- Mental clarity
- Improved focus and memory
- Increased levels of bliss
- Irresistible you!

Shopping list for everything you need:

- White basmati rice
- Split mung beans
- Spices: Coriander, cumin, fennel, fresh ginger, turmeric
- Ghee: Make your own from the Summer Recipes (or purchase at a health food store)
- Veggies: Seasonal and local veggies. Choose a diversity of colors and greens
- Sea salt or rock salt
- *Triphala*
- Herbal teas: Choose a variety of warming, cleansing seasonal teas such as ginger, lemon, licorice, cardamom, and tulsi
- Sesame oil (for self-massage)

Your Fall Cleanse Calendar

Each Day:

- Scrape your tongue.
- Drink warm water with lemon in the morning.
- Practice self-massage with sesame oil.
- Follow the Fall yoga practice.
- Consume mineral broths and herbal teas.
- Do Fall *pranayama* practice.
- Take some quiet time to yourself everyday. Follow Fall meditation practice.
- Take *triphala*.

Days 1-5

Cleanse prep: The first five days prepare you by eliminating trigger foods and foods that are acidic, clogging, and heavy, thus initiating the process of shifting your body to a more alkaline environment.

Day 1: Eliminate dairy (except ghee), alcohol, and sodas; begin taking *triphala*: 1/2 tsp in 1/2 cup warm water at night before bed.
Day 2: Eliminate sugar and animal products.
Day 3: Eliminate coffee and all processed foods.
Day 4: Eliminate all caffeine and chocolate.
Day 5: Eliminate fruit juices, dried fruit, fresh fruit, and nuts.

You are free to choose what seasonal foods you eat with the above considerations. If you need more ideas, see Fall Food Guide, and Meal Ideas and Recipes.

Days 6-10

You start to shift the body consciousness around eating and your relationship to food by introducing the mono-diet of *kichari*.

See *Tridoshic* Fall *Kichari* recipe.

Keep smiling!

Day 6: *Kichari* all meals/when hungry. To keep it interesting, add condiments and spices from your Fall Food Guide.
Day 7: *Kichari* all meals/when hungry. Wow Day 7—*keep on keeping on!*
Day 8: *Kichari* all meals/when hungry. Get creative with seasonal greens (kale, chard, spinach, collards).
Day 9: *Kichari* all meals/when hungry.
Day 10: *Kichari* all meals/when hungry. Hooray!

Days 11-14

As we have stressed before, coming out of the cleanse is as important as the cleanse itself.

Re-introduce other healthy foods but still avoid sugar, caffeine, alcohol, processed foods, chocolate, and dairy.

Chew your food well.

Avoid over-eating.

What to eat on Days 11-14?

Reintroduce a variety of grains (quinoa, barley, brown rice), healthy proteins (nuts, legumes, eggs), fruits (eaten separately from other foods) and vegetables.

How are you feeling now? Begin to bring in more variety in your diet keeping in mind your daily food practices for the Fall season.

Continue taking *triphala* up to 3 months if you suffer from indigestion, gas, bloating, or constipation.

Daily Cleanse Check-in

Day	How do you feel today? Physically, mentally, emotionally?	What is your energy level like today? (from 1, lowest, to 10, highest)	What challenges are you currently experiencing?
1			
2			
3			
4			
5			
6			
7			
8			
9			
10			
11			
12			
13			
14			

Part 6

Winter Time

Chapter 33

The Hush of Winter

"I wonder if the snow loves the trees and fields, that it kisses them so gently? And then it covers them up snug, you know, with a white quilt; and perhaps it says, "Go to sleep, darlings, till the summer comes again."

~ Lewis Carroll, *Alice's Adventures in Wonderland & Through the Looking-Glass*

Winter is the season of letting go, of endings, of decay, of death. It is the season where completion and stillness evolve naturally in preparation for what is to come. Life contracts, withdraws, and turns inside itself to reflect, hibernate, and pause.

Winter is Nature's *bardo*—the place in-between.

M

Growing up in rural Ontario, Canada allowed me to explore a Winter wonderland replete with ice-skating, snow angels, cross-country skiing, shoveling snow to get the car out of the driveway after a blizzard overnight, not to mention the occasional day off school due to snow storms. Yes!

Even though we romped through waist-high snow banks and sucked on icicles from the eaves trough, Winter was also a time to cuddle up by the fireplace, bake cookies, and come together with family and friends indoors. It was a time to nurture and hunker down. It was a time to be still (especially when the roads were closed down due to too much snow).

Ayurvedically speaking, Winter is divided into two parts. The first half of Winter relates to *vata dosha* (light, cold, dry, and changeable qualities) whereas the later part of the season is more *kapha* in nature (accentuated by qualities of damp, cold, heavy, slow, stable, and smooth). Look to the qualities of your particular climate and environment to see when the change in Winter occurs from the more *vata* expression to a more *kapha* one.

Nourish and invigorate, ground and inspire, warm and energize!

Is it not curious that Winter is the time of year in our society that we are coaxed to go out to Christmas parties, gatherings, or social events? Perhaps the calling of our wisdom body wants to be more still and inward yet we have these obligations to fulfill.

The more we ignore the inner wisdom and natural rhythms of Nature (of which we are a part), the greater the potential for imbalance, stress, and toxicity to accumulate.

Daily routine, proper foods, and lifestyle choices all contribute to boosting the immune function and balancing the nervous system to fight off those ever so common Winter blues.

Not this year honey-buns!

8 Winter Journal Questions

1. What does the Winter season represent to you?
2. What qualities are invoked within you during the Winter season?
3. What you love about the Winter time is . . .
4. What three things can you do for yourself this Winter season to stay balanced physically, mentally, and emotionally?
5. Where would you like to direct your energy this season?
6. How can you make this happen?
7. What aspect of yourself is no longer serving you that you are ready to evolve out of?
8. What aspect of yourself would you like to expand?

G & M's Winter Journals

G

*December 15*th

Something huge has shifted within me.

Not sure exactly if I can put my finger on it. A long time ago a friend said, "Just you wait, one day you will wake up and everything will just suddenly be OK."

It is not that the shift happens in a moment. It is an accumulation of the lifetimes, years, months, days and minutes of choices, practices and refinements that suddenly opens the door to grace. It means there will still be challenges and doubts. I will still feel pain. I will still be confronted with tough choices. What has shifted is the ability to navigate with confidence knowing I am responding in the most authentic way.

I recall a particular yoga practice many years ago when I was living in New York. I had been struggling with getting into handstand away from the wall for years. I always fell after a few short seconds up. I was determined and kept on practicing. That day I "suddenly" was up. Feet proudly pointing towards the ceiling, hands planted firmly on the ground. I stayed there for what seemed like forever and then gracefully came down. From then on handstand was easy.

I couldn't believe I had struggled with it for so long.

M

December 31st

December 31st, the final day of the year. Despite every moment being a new moment to reinvent myself and re-create my life, today is collectively a powerful day to let go of the old and move into the new.

Spending Christmas with my family for the first time in over a decade was amazing. As I get older I'm feeling the importance of marking these occasions and not just letting another year pass without letting those whom I love the most know it. Ram Das said, "If you think you're enlightened, go spend a week with your family."

It's so true. No matter how conscious we think we are, being with family is the place where we will be shoved up against the darkest and ugliest parts of ourselves, and asked to be completely honest with whom we are. Even though my family isn't perfect, I feel such gratitude for who they are and what they teach me. I've decided to focus on the positive and nurturing aspects of my family and accept them for who they are and the choices they make, even if they conflict with my own beliefs or values. Otherwise, I find myself coming from a limited, judgemental, and righteous place when my intention is to be more loving.

Reflecting upon the last week in Ontario, etched in my mind and heart are some beautiful moments . . . my Mom and I driving home in a snowstorm with the radio cranked, singing "Livin' On a Prayer" by Bon Jovi at the top of our lungs . . . my brother and I creating havoc on the flight from Vancouver to Toronto as we laughed and expressed our unique "Phillips family" sense of humour (which is lost on most people) . . . my Dad trying to explain to his partner's Grandson who I am. When four-year old Izzy realized that I was my Dad's daughter he paused, looked at me, and threw his arms around me with such welcome acceptance and love . . . running on the beach with the 13-year old deaf and blind dog, Finnegan, who takes the prize for an example of unconditional love.

Now it's time to shed this past year. I'm not sorry to see the back of this year as I have a feeling, a strong guttural feeling that this coming year will be the best year of my life. In fact, I've decided to make every year the best year of my life. I've decided to take 100% responsibility for my life, how it looks and feels, and how I respond to it. I've decided to be the person I can be, not the person I was in high school, or last year, or even yesterday. I've decided that I am the Master of my life and my dreams. I've decided to shimmy up nice and close to Divine Grace, and open my heart to her and surrender to the magic She brings—a life that is even more perfect then the one I thought I wanted.

Chapter 34

Winter Routines

Seasonal and Daily Practices for Winter

Stillness offered by nature to build immunity and deepen restful reflection.

Winter is here, and we start to turn inwards. Colours become pure and clean; the landscape, stark and bare. Things are stripped down as our internal fire works harder to warm us up.

In the early Winter, we gather and store, planning for the reflective weeks ahead. This is a time to slow down, to notice internal and external changes, while the body and mind prepare for the descent into darkness and the cycle of death, decay, and rebirth.

Can you feel the internal heat, the quieting of the mind, the soul beckoning you to silence? Do you notice changes in your body, mind, attitude, and routines?

Our entire being craves a Winter routine. It is during Winter that our immunity is boosted as our internal fire increases and nourishes us with a warm glow from within. Because we are set up by Mother Nature to build, strengthen, and nourish during this season, following a sound daily practice will go a long way in securing vital immunity for the year ahead. A daily practice for Winter brings the sustenance much needed and most essential for thriving within the inert nature of this season.

For those of us who are happy to slow down, it can be a meaningful transition, while for others it can feel in torturous conflict to our busy lives. Adjust we must. These practices will hold you in good stead for your lifetime.

Begin simply. Choose and set in place your routines for the day. These are your power supplies bringing you to a strong and potent place. There is a temptation to continue the activity and movement of Fall. It takes a while to allow the body to shift gears. The slowing down is an internal awareness rather than a physical stillness as we need activity to move us. It is the *yin* and *yang* of inner quietude and external motion that bring harmony in this season.

Commit to staying with the practices that work best for you. Each day we have the opportunity to create a deepening routine that will increase our life force, strengthen our immunity, and clarify our life goals so we can thrive.

1. As the Winter mornings feel like the dark of night, it may seem more challenging to wake earlier. Try to wake just before sunrise at around 7 a.m. Sunrise to mid-morning is *kapha* in quality, and your body may resist getting going, so this is a perfect time to get out of

bed and begin your morning practices to encourage flow and prevent heaviness. The main focus is to get enough rest and build the immune system. Avoid oversleeping. As always, allow yourself enough time to do your morning practices without feeling stressed or rushed.

2. Morning cleansing rituals: scrape tongue, brush teeth, start your oil pulling practice by swishing one tbsp sesame oil around the teeth and gums.

3. Once a week, gargle with a ginger/turmeric mixture (add 1/8 tsp ginger powder and 1/8 tsp turmeric to 1/2 cup warm water). This magic potion will keep your throat clear of bacteria and clear out any sticky toxins residing in the back of the throat.

4. Drink warm water with 1/2 tsp fresh grated ginger and a squeeze of lemon to assist elimination and activate digestion. Poor digestive activity in the morning accumulates toxins and leaves us feeling heavy and lethargic for the day.

5. Massage sesame oil gently in both nostrils using either a cotton bud or your baby finger to apply the oil.

6. Beautiful Body and Happy Mind Winter Practices:

    - Meditate (even five minutes is good).

    - Follow the *pranayama* practice for Winter.

    - Move (follow Winter yoga practice, dance, walk briskly, or hike). A more energized movement in Winter helps to shift stagnation and congestion and warms the body up for the day.

    - Self-massage with warm sesame oil to stimulate circulation. Take a warm shower.

    - Anoint yourself with stimulating, decongesting, and clarifying essential oils for the Winter. Choose from sage, lemongrass, ginger, grapefruit, eucalyptus, cardamom, black pepper, wintergreen, pine, juniper, myrrh, clary sage, geranium, ylang ylang, rosemary. For applications refer to aromatherapy in the Winter section.

7. Meals: Breakfast, lunch, and dinner taken at the same times each day benefit the nervous system and assist good digestion. Warming, energizing meals are best, with a focus on sweet, salty, and bitter tastes in early Winter and pungent, bitter, and astringent tastes in late Winter. Pungent herbs and warming spices enliven the digestive fire and assist metabolism. Eat away from the computer or other electronic distractions.

    - Breakfast: Light, warm, and nourishing, and ideally eaten by 10 a.m.

- Lunch: Main meal of the day and eaten around midday. Avoid over-eating. Take a short brisk walk after lunch to aid digestion.

- Dinner: Light, warming, and freshly prepared, ideally eaten by 6 p.m. Avoid heavy foods in the evening as this can result in gas, bloating, indigestion, and poor or heavy, dull sleep.

8. Before bed, take some quiet time with at least an hour of distraction-free space. Meditate, journal, pray, chant. Choose an activity that integrates your day and brings a peaceful night sleep. Getting sufficient rest is a panacea for boosting the immune system and transforming nutrients into healthy tissues. Aim for bedtime by 10 p.m.

Encourage and invite nourishment, pampering, and inner inquiry—after all, this is Winter!

Chapter 35

Winter Food Practices

Fire in the Belly

As the days grow shorter, it seems our appetites grow taller. It makes sense that we feel hungrier at this time of year. Our digestion is actually stronger in this chilly season because our *agni* is tuned to bring more heat and energy to the body just as a furnace works harder to warm our home in the Winter.

We notice that the foods that survive and thrive in the long cold Winters are the ones that sustain us. Good food practices mean good immunity, and it is in this season that we have the greatest opportunity for boosting our immune system because our bodies are deeply nourished by enhanced digestion. We have the incorrect notion that this season increases sluggishness and excess unwanted fat. It need not!

If we eat correctly, with the foods that build our bones and nourish our tissues, we will garner great immunity and fortitude for the year ahead. Avoid heaviness and congestion by eliminating heavy processed foods, junk food, rich candies, and pastries. Our food suggestions for the Winter are meant to energize the predominant elements of earth and water, and nourish air and ether. These are the building blocks of the body and mind that bring strength and a good foundation for health.

What happens to our body and mind in the Winter? From an Ayurvedic perspective, Winter is divided into early Winter and Late Winter. In early Winter, the cold, dry *vata* qualities still prevail and we need to nourish light, mobile, airy *vata* without aggravating heavy, slow, watery *kapha*. The qualities of the late season are those of the *kapha dosha*: damp, cool, smooth, slow, dense, and unctuous (slippery or greasy).

The mind can be distracted or dull if we ignore the principles of eating for the season, and the body can become sluggish, heavy, and cold. By gleaning the wisdom of Nature, we must simplify our practices for the season, and pay special attention to how we feel.

Balancing the six tastes is key in each season. In early Winter, we have a plethora of sweet root vegetables available to us: turnips, sweet potatoes, pumpkin, parsnips, carrots, cabbage. There are also the hardy bitter Winter greens such as kale and collards which grow right through the season and are widely available. These greens balance the sweet heavy root vegetables along with sweet and pungent spices of cinnamon, cardamom, ginger, cloves, black pepper, and turmeric. Spices are especially useful in this cold season to warm and energize the body. The salty taste would include sea vegetables and rock salt. Sour taste comes in the citrus fruits and stored pickles that endure through the Winter. Astringent taste is in the earth with grounding beans like chickpeas, lentils, mung beans, black beans which are particularly good in late Winter for absorbing liquids, tightening tissues and absorbing fats.

In the early Winter, we balance our bodies with the predominant sweet, sour, and salty tastes as these bring moisture, warmth, and a strong digestive fire. In the late Winter, we bring more pungent and astringent tastes to the diet. The sweet taste builds and strengthens bones and bodily tissues, boosting our immunity. Salty taste balances *vata* and the pungent taste enlivens the body and mind during the cold season.

We do need to include healthy nourishing fats in our diet. Olive oil, ghee, sesame oil, and almond oil keep the digestive fire burning. The body craves fat as it is a plentiful source of energy and warmth, as well as excellent food for the brain.

Engaging in moderation while consuming fat during Winter is the key.

Deep-fried foods or excess fats and oils can hinder digestion and clog the system so these are a no-no. Also, in the cold seasons, raw, cold foods (uncooked salads and raw vegetables, cold smoothies, drinks and juices) dampen digestion and suppress rather than strengthen the immune system.

Hot soups, stews, mineral broths, cooked whole grains, sea vegetables, fresh water fish, organic (white meat) chicken, sweet roasted root vegetables, hearty steamed greens with moderate oil dressings. These are just a few of the food ideas for Winter. The focus is: warm, nourishing, and energizing.

Tip: Avoid cold or ice-cold foods and drinks. Eliminate heavy dairy foods such as ice cream, cold milk, yoghurt, and cheese. These are all harder to digest especially in the later Winter and tend to clog the system. Winter colds are brought on and aggravated by sticky, heavy, cold foods that create mucous in the lungs and respiratory system. A hot and delicious spicy-sweet tea in the afternoon stimulates and warms the body, and alleviates sluggishness.

Tonic: Fresh ginger, lemon, and honey tea ward off colds. 1/2 inch ginger sliced, one lemon sliced, 1/2 tsp turmeric. Boil 2 cups water. Add ingredients. Turn down to simmer for 15 minutes. Add honey to sweeten (1 tsp).

Treat: See Winter Wonder Balls in Winter Recipe section.

Use the Winter Food Guide below as a guide. Eat with the season, and observe what is available at this time from farmers and local markets in your area. Get creative.

There are also several excellent Ayurvedic cookbooks that we love and recommend, which can be found in our Resource section at the back of the book.

Madhuri Phillips and Glynnis Osher

Winter Food Guide

Herb and Spice Magic for the Winter

Allspice	Anise	Asafoetida	Basil	Black Pepper
Caraway	Cardamom	Cinnamon	Cloves	Coriander
Cumin	Fennel	Garlic	Ginger	Mace
Mustard Seed	Nutmeg	Orange Peel	Oregano	Paprika
Poppy Seeds	Rosemary	Saffron	Sage	Star Anise
Thyme	Turmeric			

Winter Legumes

Aduki Beans	Black Beans	Black-Eyed Peas	Chickpeas	Lentils
Lima Beans	Mung Beans	Navy Beans	Pinto Beans	Split Peas
*Tofu	White Beans			

*In moderation

Winter Grains

Barley	Buckwheat	Corn	Millet	Oats
Pasta (soba, buckwheat, rice, rye, corn)		Quinoa	Spelt	Whole Wheat

*In moderation

Winter Fruits

Apples (stewed/cooked/raw)		Dates	Dried Fruits	Figs
Lime/Lemon/Clementines		Pears (stewed/cooked/raw)		Persimmon
Quince	Raisins			

Winter Veggies

Brussel Sprouts	Broccoli	Beets	Cabbage	Carrots
Celery	Cauliflower	Green Beans	Leeks	Onion (cooked)
Parsnip	Potato	Peppers (Orange/Red Bell)		Sweet Potatoes
Squash (All Seasonal Squash)		Salad Greens: Kale, Chard, Mustard Greens Etc. (Cooked/Steamed)		
Turnips	Yams			

Winter Dairy

Butter	*Cows Milk	Ghee	Goats Cheese/Milk

*In moderation

Winter Fish and Meat

*Beef	Eggs	Chicken (favor white meat)	*Lamb
Fish (favor fresh water fish)		Turkey (favor white meat)	Venison

Winter Nuts*, Seeds, and Condiments

Almonds	Flax Seeds	Hazelnuts	Pecans
Popcorn	Pumpkin Seeds	Sunflower	Walnuts
Pine Nuts	Sesame Seeds	Sunflower Seeds	

*Soaking your nuts in water overnight and then peeling off the skin allows for better digestion. Nuts and seeds naturally contain enzyme inhibitors, which are indigestible and therefore create toxins in the system. Only soak the amount you are going to eat that day to avoid mold and fermentation.

Winter Oils

Almond	Canola	Corn	Flax	Ghee
Olive	Mustard	Sesame	Sunflower	

*In moderation

Winter Sweeteners

Cane Sugar (unrefined)	Honey (raw is best)	*Maple syrup	Stevia

*In moderation

Winter Teas

Basil (Tulsi/Holy Basil)		Cardamom	Chai	Cinnamon
Clove	Ginger	Licorice	Orange Peel	Rosemary
Sage	*CCF (Classic Ayurvedic tea of cumin, coriander and fennel)			

*To make CCF tea take 1 tsp each of fennel seed, cumin seed, and coriander seed. Add along with 4 cups water to a small pot and bring to boil. When mixture has reached a boil, turn down to simmer for 10-15 minutes. Strain and drink. This tea is cleansing, aids the digestive system and supports the absorption of nutrients in the body while bringing the body into a state of acid/alkaline (pH) balance. A great tea to reset the body after any over-indulgences.

Winter Meal Ideas and Recipes

Breakfast: Grains are a good warming breakfast in the Winter. Add spices, seeds, nuts, and dried fruits from your Winter Food Guide for a satisfying meal to start your day off right.

- Savory breakfasts are also excellent in the morning. Add turmeric, lentils, and ginger to your grains to make for a nourishing, less-sweet breakfast.
- Experiment with your seasonal grains, or try poached, boiled, or scrambled eggs.
- Try stewed fruits with spices for a lighter breakfast.

Lunch: This is best as your main meal of the day as digestion is at its prime between noon and 2 p.m.

- Remember to include all six tastes for a balanced and satisfying meal.
- Soups, stews, and warm hearty lunches will give you the strength and support you need.
- Root veggies, Winter greens, grains, and beans or small portions of animal foods make up a good lunch!
- Experiment with a variety of foods from the Winter Food Guide.

Dinner: This can be a lighter meal taken at least three hours before bedtime.

- Enjoy a variety of spices and condiments with your meal to include all six tastes.
- Soups, light grains, small portions of animal foods, and a rotating variety of veggies are best.
- Simplicity is key for your daily evening meal.
- Eat slowly, enjoy every bite. Offer gratitude before each meal.

Spicy Winter Oats

Soak oats overnight for best digestion and absorption of nutrients.
Serves 2

3 cups water
1 cup rolled oats
1/2 tsp cinnamon
1/2 tsp ground ginger
1 tsp raisins or chopped dried figs

Toppings: cinnamon, sunflower seeds, soaked peeled almonds, and a drizzle of honey or maple syrup.

In a medium pot, bring water to a boil. Add the oats, cinnamon, ground ginger, and raisins or chopped dried figs. Cook together while stirring for three minutes if oats are pre-soaked, or eight minutes if not.

Add additional toppings as desired.

Winter Chickpea Chowder

Serves 4

Soak dried chickpeas overnight or use organic canned chickpeas.

This hearty Winter soup makes a great savory breakfast, lunch, or dinner.

8 cups water or vegetable broth
2 cups dried soaked chickpeas or 14 oz can organic chickpeas
1 tbsp olive oil
1 clove garlic
1 leek
1/2 onion
1 inch fresh peeled ginger
1 large sweet potato
1 parsnip
1 stalk celery
1/2 red bell pepper
5 leaves kale
1/2 tsp turmeric
1/2 tsp ground cumin
1/2 tsp ground coriander
1/2 tsp ground cinnamon
1/2 tsp ground nutmeg
1 tsp sea salt

1. If using dried chickpeas: soak overnight in 6 cups cold water. Throw out soaking water, and rinse beans before cooking. Do not use soaking water to cook with. Bring 6 cups water to boil, add soaked chickpeas and cook until soft—about 1 hour. A pressure cooker is a worthy kitchen investment and an invaluable friend for cooking beans in half the time. Alternatively for a quicker meal use one 14 oz can organic chickpeas.
2. Peel and dice into small pieces the garlic, onion, leeks, fresh peeled ginger, sweet potato, parsnip, celery, and red bell pepper. Wash and strip off the stalk 5 leaves of kale and tear or chop into small pieces.

3. Add 1 tbsp olive oil into a medium pot. On medium heat, sauté onions, leeks ginger, and garlic until lightly browned.
4. Add all other veggies except for the kale and sauté for a few more minutes.
5. Add 8 cups water or veggie broth and with lid on bring to a slow boil.
6. Once boiling add cooked or canned chickpeas and stir, lower to simmer for 10 minutes.
7. Add kale, turmeric, ground cumin, coriander, nutmeg and cinnamon.
8. Add salt and stir. Serve with a slice of lemon and chopped cilantro on top.
9. To make for a heartier meal, steam a variety of Winter greens with salt and ghee and add a grain from your Winter grains list.

Spice Mistress's Perky Chai

Serves 2

Afternoons are dark by 3 or 4 p.m., and we start to drag our heels. This easy Ayurvedic chai will energize *kapha* and stimulate digestion an hour or two before dinner. A rejuvenating and uplifting beverage!

3 cups water
1 inch fresh grated ginger
2 finger pinch saffron
2 finger pinch cinnamon
6 whole cloves
8 cardamom pods lightly cracked
8 black peppercorns lightly cracked
1 tsp or 1 teabag rooibos (redbush) tea/ black tea
Honey to taste
Milk or almond milk optional

Add 3 cups water to a small pot. Add ginger, cardamom, cloves, black pepper, saffron, and rooibos tea. Bring to a boil and then turn down to simmer for 10-15 minutes. Turn off heat and add the cinnamon. Stir. Add warmed or steamed milk if desired. Add honey to taste.

Take this perky chai with you in a flask so you can have it when you experience an afternoon lull.

Winter Wonder Balls

Sweet, satisfying and chock-full of nutrients!

1 cup dates
1/2 cup dried figs

1 tsp ginger powder
1/2 tsp ground cinnamon
1/2 tsp ground cardamom
2 tbsp desiccated coconut
2 tbsp cacao powder

1. Soak dates and figs for 15 minutes in boiling water until soft.
2. Remove date pits if not already pitted.
3. Strain and remove from water. Mash together well.
4. Mix in well the ginger, cinnamon, and cardamom.
5. Plop into coconut and roll into small balls.
6. Drop into cocoa powder to coat. Expect a wonderfully sticky mess!
7. Push a soaked, peeled almond into the Wonder Ball as an added treat. Indulge in moderation.

Winter Beddy-Bye Tonic

To be taken half an hour before bed.

Add a pinch of cinnamon and ground cardamom with a 1/4 tsp honey to a 1/4 cup of warm almond, whole milk or soy milk to send you off into a cozy, calm sleep.

Chapter 36

Winter Self-Care

G

My Winter landscape shifted halfway through my life. Growing up in South Africa, Winter began in June. There was no snow except for one "freak of nature" year when I was in art school and my eccentric art history teacher looked out the window and declared, "I do believe it is going to snow."

We thought she was mad as a hatter, but an hour later, sure enough, there was snow. It seems my teacher was wisely attuned to and could read Mother Nature's signs.

Now I live in North America and Winter means a high likelihood of snow. It also means extra attention to dryer cooler skin, possible weight gain, and lethargy from over-indulging in too many cozy foods and a little too much couch surfing to escape the dark, cold days.

Instead, in the Winter, we can enjoy steam saunas, hot evening baths with lung expanding oils, and gingery spicy hot tonics to satisfy and warm the body (and energize the spirit).

Winter is a beautiful opportunity for self-care. It is the season where our immunity is strengthened through rest and increased metabolic activity where we build our *ojas*. This juicy word means life-essence or vigor in Sanskrit. When our *ojas* is low and depleted, we are beginning a cycle of compromised health; when it is strong, juicy, and luscious, we are setting ourselves up for a lifetime of beauty.

Winter is the ideal season for nourishing the seven tissue layers of the body known in Sanskrit as *dhatus*. Plasma, blood, muscle, fat, bone, bone marrow/nerve, and reproductive fluid. The healthy building up of these tissues is crucial to our longevity, especially if we have become depleted through the year from disturbed metabolism, depression, mental stress, poor sleep, excessive indulgence, and general "crimes against wisdom."

Winter's seasonal depletion is only worsened by the overuse of pharmaceutical drugs and other intoxicants, and general lack of self-care. Yes, these do all add up. All these factors cause toxins to build in our body, and we need proper digestion and rest to get us back on track and to maintain and build our vitality.

Immune boosting tonics, and the correct daily routine, go a long way in assisting us with this, along with rejuvenating herbs and foods known as *rasayana*. *Ojas* is the subtle energy of the *kapha dosha* and mindful self-care is essential to nourish and nurture us so we may flower exquisitely in the Spring.

The poet Barbara Winkler describes this perfectly: "Every gardener knows that under the cloak of winter lies a miracle . . . a seed waiting to sprout, a bulb opening to the light, a bud straining to unfurl. And the anticipation nurtures our dream."

Our dream is perfect balance and health so we may fulfill our purpose here as we were meant to. The rhythm of the Winter season is slow and soft and the most vital thing we can observe is the one thing that sometimes may seem inaccessible.

Inner Stillness.

We must take time each day to nurture this quietude. The nourishing self-care practices we take on for the season reward us with the gift of health and longevity. These practices focus on warmth, sweetness, comfort, being, and allowing.

There is nothing more nurturing for body, mind, and soul than a quiet aromatic evening bath or morning shower with salt scrubs and expansive aromatic oils, and nothing more satisfying than an afternoon uplifting tonic with fragrant ginger, feisty lemon, and tonifying honey, sipped on to keep the body warm and the spirit bright.

Choose two or three of these soul-care suggestions that resonate with you and establish these practices, rotating them consistently in your daily Winter routine.

Ojas for Life Winter Face Cleanse

Put your best Winter face forward. Our face needs protection to endure the harsh cold conditions. Ground grains, nuts, and milk are the ideal ingredients for a smooth, moon-like skin.

Make enough for a week or two supply of this energizing cleanser for a vital, bright, and well-nourished complexion. Nuts, grains, and milks are full of nourishment and are akin to a balanced nutrient-rich breakfast for your skin!

Dry ingredients

1 cup barley, ground into a powder in an electric grinder (or mortar and pestle, if you like)
1/4 cup almond meal (finely ground almonds)
1/4 cup dried ground orange peel
1/4 cup dried milk powder
(Blend together, store in an airtight glass jar in a cool dry place or in the refrigerator)

Wet ingredients

Warm water
Lemongrass or lemon essential oil
(Add to dry mix and make into a paste for each cleansing application)

For your daily morning face cleansing ritual, take a tbsp of the dry mixture and add warm water and one drop lemongrass or lemon essential oil as needed to give the mixture a creamy, thick consistency. Mix into a paste, and with upward sweeping and circular strokes, massage over entire neck and face. Without scrubbing, gently massage face all over with this enlivening cleanser. Wash off with warm water, and gently pat skin dry with a clean towel.

Guardian of the Skin Winter Moisturizer

Make enough for a week or two supply of this rich moisturizer for bright, nourished skin. Use in the morning to moisturize and protect your skin for the day.

Mix well together and store in an airtight glass bottle:

1 cup unrefined almond oil
12 drops lemongrass EO
12 drops lavender EO
3 drops rosemary EO
1/4 tsp honey

1 bottle of witch hazel toner to have on hand.
(Do not mix into oil blend; keep separate)

Each morning after cleansing, take 1/2 tsp of oil blend and mix with 1 tsp witch hazel toner and massage into face. Use more oil blend if needed.

Alive Winter Bath Salt Scrub

Make enough for a week or two supply of this lung-expanding, skin rejuvenating, aromatic body scrub. Rich in minerals, oils, and aromatic wisdom to wake up and warm sluggish, cold skin.

4 cups coarse sea salt
1/2 cup sesame oil
1/2 cup olive oil
6 drops pine or fir EO
6 drops lemongrass EO

4 drops eucalyptus or ginger EO
4 drops rosemary EO

Stir salts, oils and essential oils to richly and lavishly coat the salt grains. Place in a sealed glass jar and keep on hand near the shower so that you can grab the mix whenever your skin needs a pick-me-up.

Tip: Stand in shower. Wet skin. Turn off water, or step away from the water flow. Grab a handful of the oily salts and lightly scrub all over body. Turn water back on and rinse. The body will have a thin coating of the oils and feel soft and supple all day. Treat yourself to this at least once a week in the mornings!

Hibernation Bath Soak

Mmmmmm, a soothing bath at the end of a frosty day! Add some joy to your bathwater and embrace yourself with a fragrant soak before bed to ensure a restful sleep. The minerals absorb into your skin and replenish your body. Make enough for about four baths.

1 cup Epsom salts
1 cup sea salt
5 drops clary sage or frankincense EO
5 drops ginger EO
5 drops fir or cedar or juniper EO

Mix together and store in airtight glass jar. Use 1/2 cup aromatic salt soak in each bath. Sweet dreams as your lymphatic system works freely and your lungs are open and clear!

Winter Aromatherapy

Every season brings an opportunity to benefit from the healing plant essences. In the Winter, we use essential oils to balance the cold, heavy, damp qualities of the season that can affect our body and make us feel sluggish, depressed, and congested. Aromatherapy energizes the mind, enlivens the emotions, and can elevate your spirits even on the darkest days. It is a powerful healing tool to stimulate and rejuvenate the system, and boost immunity.

Slowly build your aromatherapy apothecary for each season, and you will always have a remedy on hand.

The oils are versatile and can be blended in a multitude of ways.

Suggested Essential Oil List for Winter
(Uplifting, energizing, decongesting, pungent, strengthening)

Stock your bathroom apothecary with at least three or four of these fragrant friends: ginger, cardamom, eucalyptus, rosemary, clove, cinnamon, black pepper, frankincense, clary sage, cedar, pine, juniper, basil, lemongrass, lemon, grapefruit, geranium, lavender, and cypress.

How to apply aromatherapy to your daily Winter practice:

Make a pure essential oil blend using two or three different oils. Store in a dark glass airtight bottle. You can also keep four or five different essential oils in your bathroom cabinet and blend as needed, or use individually as preferred.

1. Massage oil: By adding an essential oil blend to a carrier oil you can have a customized massage blend on hand to use as needed. Two lovely massage carrier oils for the Winter are sunflower or almond oil or an equal mix of the two. A ratio of 48-90 drops of pure essential oil to 4 oz carrier oil is the standard range depending on how potent you want your blend. Keep your blend simple when starting out, using only three or four essential oils. Play and experiment as you discover the best scents for you.

2. Bath oil: The best way to use essential oils in the bath is to mix them with salts or an emulsifier such as milk or your carrier oil. You can also add your custom massage blend directly into the bath. Two to three tablespoons makes for a luxurious bath and allows the oils to be absorbed deeply into the skin.

A good ratio is 10-20 drops essential oil mixed with 1/2 cup of salt or emulsifier.

Aromatic baths in the Winter are excellent for the circulatory system, respiratory system, and for rejuvenating the entire immune system.

3. Direct Palm Inhalation: Apply 1-2 drops of your favourite essential oils to your palms, rub together gently, and inhale deeply. This is an excellent method of use for a quick and easy exposure to the essential oils.

4. Facial steam: Place 1-3 drops in steaming hot water in a bowl, cover head with a towel, steam face. Excellent for opening sinuses and clearing stagnation. Eucalyptus, basil, lemon, and ginger are particularly good at this time of year.

G & M's Winter Journals

G

February 21st

This morning, on the day of the new moon in February, I was driving to my studio and feeling somewhat blue. Depressed really. I am so intent on being positive and cheerful that revealing anything different out loud makes me feel totally exposed. This is my pitta *perfectionism and inner-critic. You know . . . the one that makes me suffer the most!*

My father was manic-depressive, and in those earlier days nobody understood or acknowledged what that was. Any mental illness was taboo and hush-hushed. We never spoke about it in "public."

I have often feared in my darkest moments that I inherited a piece of my father's illness through strands of ancestral DNA. Depression is a condition that can stop you in your tracks and make you feel as if there is nothing worth doing or living for.

Most often the first step to recovery is admitting there is a problem but still the shame and the stigma society has placed on "mental illness" has rendered us silent. I believe that had my father the freedom to explore his deep-rooted mental/emotional suffering, his life story would have had a different and happier ending. His desperation compelled him to attempt to end his life by jumping in front of a bus. I was 12 years old. With severe injury to his brain, he spent the balance of his life in a mental institution and died sadly alone. This tragedy shaped our family and also gave us profound resilience and courage.

Sadly there are an escalating number of people who are suffering from mental illness and our medical healthcare system is for the most part at a sorry loss. Western sciences see the mind and body as separate and so treatments are given from that perspective. Ayurvedic psychology views the mind and the body as one. The mind is a reflection of the body and the body a mirror of the mind. There is an understanding here that both are expressions of consciousness.

This gives me great hope. Ayurvedic sciences have uncovered the power of simple daily lifestyle practices, self-care, and spiritual therapies such as mantra, prayer, yoga, and meditation, to bring balance and peace to the mind.

The path of Ayurveda is a journey into our own Being to remind us we are Love. Through this profound path we can smooth the sharp edges of mental suffering. I have experienced this in my own life and I am grateful.

I reflect on the miraculous healing that can come from just a small shift in consciousness and as I finally arrive at my studio a divinely-timed email with my horoscope for the week confirms: "This new moon can bring a powerful emotional healing, but we have to start by acknowledging our wounds and reaching for the faith that these wounds—like all wounds—can be healed."

Yes, they can.

M

February 23rd

What If?

What if everything is okay?
What if the universe always has my best interest at heart?
What if there really is nothing wrong?
What if struggle wasn't a personal requirement?
What if I saw the beauty more and the so-called "problems" less?
What if I lived from a place of love no matter what?
What if I allow myself to just be?
What if I can't get it wrong?
What if my life matters more then I'll ever know?
What if love is the most powerful force there is?
What if I didn't underestimate my divinity and perfection?
What if I embraced life entirely?

What if it really is a miracle?

You,
me,
this day,
this breath.

Chapter 37

Winter Yoga, *Pranayama*, and Meditation Practices

Yoga: Light Your Inner Hearth

Use your Winter yoga flow to inspire, rejuvenate, and rebalance. Nourish yourself during this natural time of hibernation, while energizing your system to warm up and keep a jolly spring in your step. The fruits of a consistent daily practice are bountiful. Your immune system will be fortified, and the Winter doldrums will be kept at bay.

To reduce both *vata* and *kapha* at this time of year, practice your yoga in a steady, nourishing, and energizing way.

Most importantly, listen to your body and the wisdom it is imparting on any given day.

> **Winter Flow Tips**
> ~ Practice at the same time every day to generate routine.
> ~ Be consistent.
> ~ Ideal time to practice: mornings, between sunrise and 10 a.m.
> ~ Anytime is better than not at all.
> ~ Manage your energy with calm and steady breathing, in and out through your nose, or use *ujjayi* breath throughout your practice as described below.

Yoga Time

This practice is wonderful to do in the morning to prepare you physically and mentally for your day. It takes just 20 minutes. Feel free to take longer in each posture if you have the time. Some yoga is better than no yoga. Set your morning alarm so you can rise and shine!

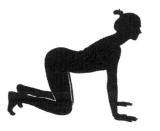 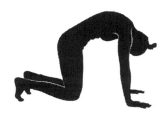

1. The Cat's Meow (*Marjariasana*: Cat Stretch)
(1-2 min.)
Come onto your hands and knees, placing your wrists directly under your shoulders and your knees directly under your hips. As you take a long, slow, and steady inhalation, tip your tailbone towards the sky, drop your belly towards the earth, and sequentially lift up your chest and then head. As you take a calm and steady breath out, curl your tailbone towards the floor, lift your navel skyward, and relax your neck and head to the ground. Repeat 5X.

2. Thread the Needle
(1 min. each side)
Stay on all fours from the previous posture. Slide the back of your right hand and arm along the floor behind your left hand far enough so that your right shoulder gently rests on the floor. Relax here. Keep some weight in your left hand for the most support or you may extend your left hand up towards the ceiling. Breathe slowly and deeply (if you feel any discomfort in the head or neck, come out of the posture. Your body weight is more on the shoulder, not on the neck). Press into your left hand for support to return to the starting position.
Repeat on the 2nd side.

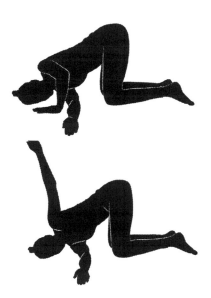

3. Mr. Cobra (*Bhujangasana*: Cobra)
(1 min.)
Come down onto your belly with your legs straight out behind you.

The first variation of this posture (for those with sensitive low backs or previous back injury) is to come into "Sphinx" where your forearms are placed flat on the floor and your upper arms are at a 90 degree angle. Place your focus at your lower back and breathe slowly and deeply.

The deeper variation of this posture, "Cobra" (if you have a healthy back) is to place your hands underneath your shoulders on the floor. Inhale and begin to lift your head and chest off of the floor to a comfortable degree. Stay here and breathe into your lower back area for 5-10 breaths. Repeat.

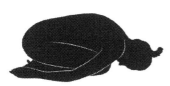

4. Child's Pose...aaaaaawh (*Balasana*: Pose of the Child)
(1 min.)
Press your buttocks back to sit on your heels, resting your forehead on the ground (if your buttocks do not rest on your heels, place a pillow or folded blanket in between buttocks and heels so that you can relax). Bring your arms by your sides, palms upwards with the elbows slightly bent. Breathe slowly and deeply into the belly 5-10X.

5. Squat...come on-give it a try! (*Namaskarasana*: Squat)
(1 min.)
This grounding practice will open your hips and increase flexibility. If you have knee problems (or pain in any joint while doing this), skip this practice. Place your feet at least hip distance apart with your toes slightly turned out. If your heels don't touch the floor naturally, place a folded up blanket underneath your heels so that you can relax your ankles. Press your palms together. Breath down into your hips and lower back area. Stay here for 5-10 breaths. To come out, place your hands on the floor in front of you, tip your bottom-end towards the sky, and ta-da, you're in the next posture…

6. Bottoms Up (*Uttanasana*: Forward Fold)
(1 min.)
In this forward fold have your feet parallel and apart 6-10 inches. Bend your knees until your belly button and thighs touch. Relax your head, neck, and jaw. Breathe into your lower back area, and let go of any accumulated tension.

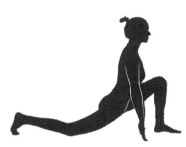

7. Lovin' Lungin' (Lunge)
(1 min. each side)
From your forward fold, step your right foot all the way back until your left knee is directly over your left ankle. Place your right knee down. Place your fingertips on the ground beside your heel; otherwise, place your hands on your thigh. Keep scooping your heart up towards the sky to create the feeling of a mini back bend (opposed to rounding/curving your spine). Stay for 5-10 breaths before switching to the second side.

8. Down doggie, down (*Adho Mukha Svanasana*: Downward Facing Dog)
(1 min.)
From your lunge, step your right foot back so that both of your hands are pressing into the floor, feet are parallel, hip distance apart, and your sitting bones are pointing up towards the sky. Keep your head in line with your spine and breeeeeeeeathe!

Transition: walk your feet forward until they are in between your hands and you are in another forward fold. Gradually roll your body up sequentially through your spine until you are standing upright.

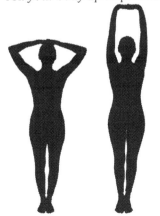

9. Dynamic Tree (*Tadasana*: Palm Tree)
(1 min.)
Stand with your feet, knees, and thighs together. Interlace your fingers together and rest the knuckles on the top of your head so the palms are facing the ceiling. On an inhalation, rise up to the balls of your feet and simultaneously lift your palms towards the ceiling. Hold for a moment before exhaling and lowering your heels to the floor and hands to the head. Repeat this six more times.

10. Wheeeeeeee! (*Kati Chakrasana*: Waist Rotating Pose)
(1 min.)
Stand with your feet at least shoulder width apart. Begin to spiral your torso to your right and wrap your right arm behind you as your left arm comes across the front of your body. Keep your elbows bent. Now, do this in the opposite direction. Begin to gather some momentum, swinging the arms around the torso, and gently touching the kidneys as your arms wrap around to the back. Carry on with this dynamic posture for approximately 1 minute. Breathe naturally as you move in this posture.

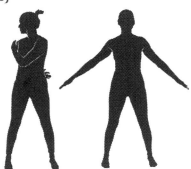

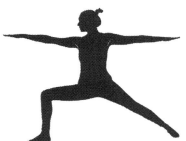

11. Warrior Deux (*Viribhadrasana* Two: Warrior Two)
(2 min.)
Start by standing with both feet together. Take the left leg back approximately 3-4 feet and place the left foot on a forward angle of about 45 degrees. Inhale—raise both arms up to shoulder height. Exhale—bend your right knee until it is in line with your right ankle. Press into the back edge of your left foot to feel the power through your legs. Look towards the middle finger of your right hand. Breathe here for 5 full breaths. Inhale to press into your feet, engage your abdominal muscles, and return upright.
Repeat on the second side.

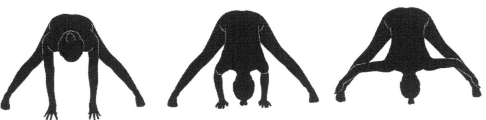

12. Hurts So Good (*Prasarit Padottanasana*: Wide Leg Forward Fold)
(2 min.)
Have your feet in a wide stance to begin, with your toes turned slightly inward. Place your hands on your hips. Inhale—make your spine as long as you can. Exhale—and fold forward from your waist until your torso is parallel to the floor. Stay here for 5 breaths. Exhale and let your head and upper back relax forward towards the ground. Place your hands on the floor where they are comfortable. Stay for 5 breaths. To come back up, place your hands on your hips, engage your abdominal muscles, and inhale to return to standing.

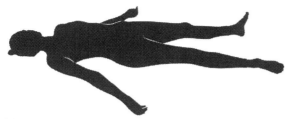

13. Icing on the Cake (*Savasana*—Corpse Pose)
(5-10 min.)
Savasana is the most coveted practice as it is the posture that restores the nervous system and gives us time to integrate everything we have done in our practice. *Savasana* is the *ojas*—the sustenance, immunity, and vitality of our yoga practice!

Lay down on your back with your head and spine straight, legs apart, letting the feet flop out to the sides. Arms are away from the sides of the body slightly and the palms face upward (use a bolster under the knees if your lower back is sore. Cover up with a blanket to stay warm if needed). Close your eyes.

Let your entire body relax. Begin at your toes and relax your feet. Move your awareness up through the body all the way to the head, consciously letting go of any stress or tension along the way. The breath is completely natural. Surrender into the stillness and silence of this posture.

Once you have completed the practice, start to wiggle your fingers and toes. Stretch your body in any way that feels wonderful!

Roll to one side and use your hands to push you to an upright position.

In-JOY-ment!

- Notice how you are feeling. How has this simple yoga practice transformed your body and mind?

- Before jumping up and carrying on with your day, take a moment to smile. Send your smile down into your toes, legs, and pelvis. Smile down into your organs: your spleen, liver, lungs, and heart. Allow your smile to spread to every cell of your body and tap into your inner In-JOY-ment!

- Commit to allowing joy to move through you today (and everyday).

- Commit to feeling light and joyful.

- Commit to smiling at the people you meet today and spreading a little joy around.

Winter Breathing: Bring on Darth Vader

The beauty of all of the various *pranayama* practices within yoga is that you can affect your body and mind, and redirect energy through the conscious awareness and manipulation of the breath.

Once you have learned and practiced various *pranayama* techniques, you will be able to discern which practices are beneficial for you at different times, depending on what effect you are seeking. The time of day, season, body temperature, and state of your mind and emotions are all things to consider when choosing your *pranayama* practice *du jour*.

Ujjayi is the victorious breath. This conscious breathing technique is wonderful to do during the long dark days of Winter, for if you can make it through this season and still be sane, you certainly are victorious. We are not sure if that is why the ancient Yogis gave it this name 5,000 years ago or not, but we have a sneaking suspicion that they too got the Winter blues at times.

Ujjayi can help to sooth any sorry state of mind, increase your focus so you have the wherewithal of a Jedi Knight, and relax your nervous system to the point where you feel you have just had a trip to the spa. *Ujjayi* has also been translated as the psychic breath. If you get really good at it, you can begin to read your co-workers minds at the office (these are the great benefits of yogic practice).

This technique helps to relieve insomnia, calms the nervous system, and benefits those with high blood pressure. I find that *ujjayi* is heating in quality yet very balancing. It is a breath that you can incorporate into your *asana* (posture) practice to help keep the mind focused.

The How-To of *Ujjayi* Breathing

1. Sit in a comfortable position, in a chair or cross-legged; wherever you can have an elongated spine.

2. Establish a slow, calm, and steady breathing pattern in and out through your nostrils.

3. Take a deep breath in and as you exhale, whisper the sound, "haaaaaaaaaaa," out loud (like you're breathing down someone's neck. Think Darth Vader in *Star Wars*). Feel how that generates a slight constriction at the back of the throat (glottis).

4. Do the same thing again but this time whisper, "ha," with your mouth closed, again feeling the constriction at the back of the throat.

5. If that feels easy and comfortable for you, keep the constriction of the glottis and inhale with the mouth closed. Imagine you are sipping the breath in and out through the throat.

6. Continue to inhale and exhale with the constriction of the glottis and an audible sound (like Darth Vader, a baby snoring, or the sound of the ocean).

7. Carry on with this practice for 5-20 minutes.

Practice Tips

- The sound of the *ujjayi* breath is audible yet not at all strained or forced.

- The more refined you become in the practice of this *pranayama*, the subtler the breath will be.

Winter Meditation: Seeing and Being. The Power is Within You

In the dark depths of this season, it is easy to succumb to the dreariness that envelops our mind, especially in cities with shorter days and rainy weather, where it is often easy to forget that the Sun exists in our solar system. Days or weeks may go by without any sunlight, the sky gets lower, and the clouds are suffocating; squeezing out that cheery, positive outlook that comes naturally in the Summer months.

So, how to look on the bright side?

The external environment has an impact on us, without a doubt. However, cultivating a deeper relationship to our own mental and emotional state where we are not whisked away by the whims of the weather, other people, or anything external is the mastery of our own internal environment (and our life).

The creative power of visualization should not be underestimated.

By focusing the mind and activating our emotional body, we can have a positive impact on restructuring the chemical make-up of the brain, our perceptions, and the cellular make-up of the body. This is how we can be our own healer. By imagining light energy or *prana* moving into the areas of the body that need healing, we literally rebuild new neuro-pathways that create new ways of seeing and being.

The How-To of the Healing Light Visualization

1. Find a comfortable place to sit with your spine straight (in a chair, with your back against a wall, or cross-legged).

2. Place your hands face up on your thighs (to uplift your energy) or in *Chin Mudra* with your index finger curled in to touch the root of the thumb, palms up.

3. Close your eyes. Scan through your entire body with your awareness. Notice any areas in the body where you may be holding tension and invite these places to relax (you can mentally say "relax" to the various body parts as you let go of any tension or tightness).

4. Let your breath be natural and easy.

5. Bring your awareness to your heart centre. Imagine a tiny light or candle flame residing in your heart. As you inhale, visualize the light of this flame radiating out in all directions through your body. As you exhale—relax. On the next inhalation, see the light growing larger and brighter filling up more space of your body. As you exhale—relax.

6. Continue to inhale and see the light expanding and illuminating your entire body. Relax as you exhale. With every inhalation see the light moving out further and further until your entire body is surrounded with this golden light energy, removing any blockages, tension, or contraction in the mind and body.

7. Visualize the light filling the room you are in . . . your home . . . your neighbourhood . . . your city . . . your country . . . the whole planet.

8. Continue to breathe naturally, and bathe in the healing light energy. Stay here for at least 10 breaths (or as long as you wish).

9. Bring your attention back to the source—your own heart. Notice how you are feeling now, physically, mentally, and emotionally.

10. When you feel ready take three deep, cleansing breaths in and out through the nose. Place your hands in *Pranam Mudra* with your palms touching in front of your heart, and take a moment to consciously acknowledge any benefits or transformation you are experiencing.

11. Know that you can return to this state at any time you choose.

Practice Tip

Practice this visualization from a place of possibility. Trust in your own capacity to relax and heal through your own creative imagination just as children do.

Chapter 38

Winter Ceremony and Ritual

Winter is a sublime time for ritual. In many ways, we go deep into the silence of the season and naturally we retreat into the warmth of our homes and hearts. The holidays give pause for many cultures to celebrate and honour their spiritual roots. We can truly take advantage of this cold, dark season to investigate the world within ourselves.

One of the rituals that so many of us love in the Wintertime is gathering with friends and deepening relationships (preferably near a cozy fireplace). It seems the quiet, contemplative energy of the season invites reflective, insightful conversations and profound connections.

Two thirds of the way through December comes the Winter Solstice, a great time of symbolism and power, with the Sun being at its southernmost point in the sky. This moment marks the beginning of the Winter and the longest night and shortest day of the year. We are slowly ascending back into the light as the days grow longer after the Solstice.

As the daylight hours increase, so does an increase in positive energy flow into our lives. The second half of Winter is a brilliant time to contemplate the idea of death and rebirth. Winter is a season of decay and dying. We witness this in the bare trees, the stark landscapes, and even in the stripped down silence of our mind.

How spectacular is Nature preparing the way for creation and allowing us the opportunity to start again each year? These are the cycles of birth and death, elation and dismay, strength and weakness, health and sickness, prosperity and poverty. This time of the year is the revolution of change where we can surrender to our inner shadow and move freely into the light.

From an Ayurvedic perspective, the Winter season is the prime time to build *ojas*. As we have written previously, this juicy word means immunity, vitality, or life force. Because *ojas* is built when we slow down and bring peace and presence into our mind, body, and soul, Winter Solstice marks the beginning of this profound opportunity to fortify ourselves and boost our strength.

These Winter rituals are performed for strengthening immunity as we take reflection:

- To share our love with friends and nourish relationships by slowing down and going deeper.
- To move confidently through the darkness into the light.
- To celebrate the cycles of our existence and connection with Natures cycles.
- To soften, integrate, understand, expand, strengthen, and build a foundation of health.

Your Irresistible Life

- To strengthen our trust in endings and beginnings.

In China, the Solstice (or "Extreme Winter") is celebrated with the *Dongzhi* Festival on or around December 21st, when sunshine is weakest and daylight shortest. The origins of this festival can be traced back to the *yin* and *yang* philosophy of balance and harmony in the Cosmos.

Following this moment, the longer daylight hours mean an increase in positive energy flowing in. The philosophical significance of this is symbolized by the *I Ching* (The Book of Change), inside of which there is a hexagram *fù* which symbolizes "Returning," and is linked with the month of the Winter Solstice.

The lines of change here symbolize the idea of a turning point—the time of darkness has past. The days that follow the Winter Solstice bring the gift of light. After a time of decay comes that turning point. The powerful light returns. There is movement, but it is not brought about by force. The movement is natural, arising spontaneously.

For this reason, the transformation of the old becomes easy. The old is discarded and the new is introduced. The movement is cyclic, and the course completes itself. Therefore it is not necessary to hasten anything artificially. We learn to trust that everything comes of itself at the appointed time.

This particularly syncopated point in time is, literally and figuratively, the meeting of Heaven and Earth.

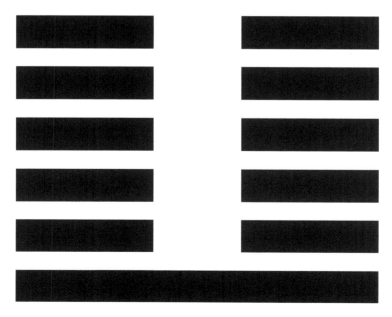

Winter Ceremony Themes: Darkness to Light, *Yin/Yang*, Endings and Beginnings

Create your Winter sacred space with some of the following things, be they images or actual objects: stars, snowflake mandalas, ice, darkness, light, etc.

Remove all of the Fall objects from your altar, and place a new cloth or covering and other meaningful items to mark the season. Light a candle, sit in contemplation, and visualize moving through the darkness and into the light.

Winter rituals inspire us to set our dreams in motion. Create a vision board for your dream. Perhaps use the hexagram *fù* symbol as a starting point. Gather images, words, ideas, and paste them onto a board or in your journal. Expand the vision of your life, bringing more meaning and potency to your actions. Describe what you feel, what you see, and place this in your sacred space.

As a sacred environment that is set up and energized with your intentions, your altar acts as the witness, holding the space for your ceremonies and rituals. Once you have set up your personal space for ritual you may find that small miracles begin to happen. Awakenings may spark new ideas, feelings of joy, and motivation.

If you have not already set up your altar space, now is a good time to do so.

Chapter 39

Winter Restoration: *Rasayana*

5-Day Rejuvenation to Build Immunity and Nourish *Ojas*

"What good is the warmth of summer, without the cold of winter to give it sweetness."

~ John Steinbeck, *Travels with Charley: In Search of America*

Why a Rejuvenating *Rasayana* Winter Practice?

At this time of year, we need to build our immunity, our life force, and go inward to nourish ourselves on a deep level. We welcome in the sweet things in life, as the sweet taste is anabolic—strengthening, stabilizing, happy-making, and increases *ojas*.

Ojas is the essence of our life-sap, the nectar of our existence. Five days of focused self-love enhances our connection to our most sensual and intimate self. This is a 5-Day inner retreat to re-spark your warmest desires.

Rasayana, or rejuvenation therapy, is one of the eight branches of Ayurveda. *Rasa* in Sanskrit means: nectar, essence, or flavor; and *ayana* means path. Therefore, *rasayana* means: The path of essence.

This ancient practice of rejuvenation nourishes body, boosts immunity, and helps to keep the mind in good health. The main goal of Ayurvedic rejuvenation or *rasayana* therapy is to restore spirit and vitality.

Enjoy these delicious foods, treats, and practices to pamper yourself.

The Benefits to You:

- Nourishment for your life force
- Increased immunity
- Glowing skin
- Increased energy and strength
- Increased oxytocin/endorphins (the feel-good hormone)
- Self-love
- Increased sexy you
- Increased sensuality
- Bliss through the roof!

Pre-rejuvenation preparation: The night before you begin, soak 10 almonds in water and then continue to do this every evening in preparation for eating them the following morning.

Food guidelines for your 5-Day Rejuvenation:

Eliminate all refined sugar, caffeine, processed foods, sodas, animal foods, alcohol, pastries, breads, cheese, deep fried foods, cold cereals, and cold drinks.

Choose organic foods when possible. Follow recipes in the Winter Food Guide and create your own simple, nourishing meals from the lists provided.

Your Winter Rejuvenation Calendar

Days 1-5

- Daily *abhyanga* self-massage with sesame oil.
- Continue with your daily Winter yoga and *pranayama* practice.
- Aromatherapy practice: Morning steam with essential oils of rosemary, eucalyptus, or lavender. Add 4 cups boiled water to a stainless steel bowl. Add a total of three drops of essential oil. Cover head and bowl with a towel while leaning over and inhaling deeply. Three to five minutes will do the trick.
- Eat 10 soaked and peeled almonds before breakfast.
- Ayurvedic Oatmeal for breakfast (See Winter Meal Ideas and Recipes).
- Sip herbal teas throughout the day.
- Choose any of the Winter recipes for meals with a focus on sweet, warm, and nourishing.
- Winter Wonder Balls: Have one a day for five days, reminding you of the natural sweetness of life (See Winter Meal Ideas and Recipes).
- Repeat mentally 10 times "I inhale love and abundance. I exhale peace and gratitude."
- Gratitude Journal: Write a list of at least 20 things you are grateful for.
- Drink 1/2 cup of warmed milk before bed (organic cows/almond/rice/oat) with a pinch of nutmeg.

Shopping List for Everything You Need:

- Ghee
- Dates
- Dried figs
- Oats
- Honey
- Milk (your choice, organic if possible)
- Almonds
- Dried coconut

- Cocoa powder
- Sesame oil for self-massage
- Spices: ginger powder (fresh/ground), ground cinnamon, ground cardamom, desiccated coconut, nutmeg, cardamom, saffron
- Essential oils: rosemary, eucalyptus, geranium, or lavender

Daily Cleanse Check-in

Day	How do you feel today? Physically, mentally, emotionally?	What is your energy level like today? (from 1, lowest, to 10, highest)	What challenges are you currently experiencing?
1			
2			
3			
4			
5			

Part 7

Going Deeper

Chapter 40

Weird Ayurvedic Practices . . . That Work!

Neti Pot (*Jala Neti*): Nasal Cleansing with Salt Water

Nasal cleansing with salt water is a fantastic practice to remove mucous and congestion from the nasal cavities and clear your sinuses. This practice may be beneficial for those with asthma, allergies, headaches, fogginess in the mind, depression, colds, hay fever, tonsillitis, and other disorders of the throat, ears, and eyes.

Contra-indications: chronic bleeding in the nose; excessive dryness of the nostrils; and/or those with a structural block such as deviated septum.

How to nasal cleanse: Buy a *neti* pot. Prepare 1 1/2 cups of body temperature water and thoroughly dissolve 1/2 tsp of salt into the water. You may need to adjust the proportions, however, the key is to have the osmotic pressure of the water balanced with those of the body fluids so that there is no irritation of the mucous membranes in the sinus cavities.

Once your warm salt water is ready in your *neti* pot, stand over the sink, place the tip of the *neti* pot spout in the nostril that is more open or has a greater flow of breath moving through it. Tilt your head to the side, breathe through your mouth, and allow the saline solution to flow in through one nostril and out the other. If the water goes down your throat, you do not have the proper positioning of your head and may be tilting the head back too far.

When half of the water has passed through the nostrils, stop, blow the nose gently if there is extraneous mucous, and then repeat the process with the other nostril until you have used up all of the water in your pot. After completing this you must dry your nostrils properly to avoid trapped water in the sinuses.

To dry your nostrils, close the right nostril with your thumb, inhale and exhale quickly in a rhythmic way, emphasizing the exhalation, 10-20 times. Repeat with the other nostril. Do the same breathing with both nostrils open, 10-20 times.

If you still feel like water is stuck in the nostrils, start from a standing position with feet four feet apart, bend forward from the waist until your torso is at a 45 degree angle, and face looking at the floor (not back behind you). Let the water drain out here and then stand up and repeat the breathing practice from above to dry the nostrils. Ever so gently, use a tissue to blow the nose if there is any remaining mucous or water.

Do not blow the nose too hard at any time during this practice as water could be pushed into the ears.

Nasya: Nasal Administration of Medicated Oil or Ghee

Nasya is one of the practices done in the classic *Panchakarma* (Five Actions Ayurvedic Cleanse) and can also be used as a stand alone therapy that is fantastic to lubricate dry nostrils, improve immunity, ward off foreign invaders trying to get into the body through the nostrils, reduce headaches, migraine, calm the mind, and assist most problems from the shoulders up: ear, eye, throat, and jaw.

How to nasally administer oil or ghee: Purchase a good quality medicated herbal *nasya* oil or simply use organic ghee or other oil appropriate for your *dosha*. Place two drops of oil or a little bit of ghee on your pinky finger (with trimmed nails of course) and gently insert your little finger into your nostril, massaging the inner rim of the nostril. Sniff dramatically to draw the oil upward into the sinuses. Repeat with the other nostril.

Tongue Scraping

This is definitely one of the best investments of your time to improve your health. If you have been reluctant to do or try anything Ayurvedic, try this. Tongue scraping will clear off the toxic gunk and bacteria (*ama*) that is on your tongue when you wake up in the morning. It reduces halitosis, improves oral and digestive health, and stimulates the internal organs. The best thing is that it only takes seconds of your time to do.

How to scrape your tongue: Buy a stainless steel tongue scraper. First thing in the morning and before you drink anything, take your tongue scraper and starting at the back of the tongue, gently pull the tongue scraper forward, clearing off any coating. Do this 5-10 times, depending on the amount of *ama* (coating). Be sure not to either start so far back on the tongue that you gag, or be too aggressive with your scraping.

Oil Pulling

Another simple, yet profoundly effective, practice that involves swishing oil around in your mouth, subsequently pulling out toxins from the saliva, and reducing bacteria, fungus and other organisms from the mouth, gums, and teeth. The benefits are numerous and expand beyond the mouth: strengthens the teeth, gums, and jaw, prevents halitosis, cavities, and gingivitis, decreases pain in the jaw, tongue, and ears, reduces headaches, clears sinus congestion, helps with insomnia, and decreases allergies, just to name a few.

How to: Take 1 tbsp of cold-pressed organic sesame or coconut oil, swish it around in your mouth for 10-15 minutes, and then spit out the oil.

Chapter 41

Ayurvedic Home Remedies

These remedies are by no means a substitute for the advice of your personal health care practitioner.

OK, we have to say that for legal reasons, however the ideal scenario is that you do become your own best healer. What do we mean?

Prevention, prevention, prevention!

This book is designed to walk you through the steps to assist you in aligning with the flow of Nature and the natural rhythms of the seasons. Getting deeply connected to your body through paying attention, listening, understanding, and then responding is the doorway into a life of great health.

Yes, we all get sick every now and then. Do not ignore the symptoms that your body is desperately trying to communicate to you. Try these suggestions and, of course, when in doubt, please do get the help you need from your health care practitioner.

Achy joints

If your joints are popping and cracking and feel dry and stiff:

Remedy 1—Avoid cold, dry foods and nightshades such as potatoes, eggplant, and tomatoes.

Remedy 2—Ginger/castor oil pack. Pour 2 tbsp castor oil onto a cotton cloth/facecloth and add 4 drops ginger essential oil. Place over specific areas of pain for at least 15 minutes while lying in relaxation pose.

Remedy 3—Daily intake of curcuma (turmeric powder) by taking 1/2 tsp turmeric in warm milk or warm water twice daily.

Remedy 4—Gentle daily yoga postures after a warm sesame oil self-massage.

If your joints are painful, inflamed, feel hot and skin looks flushed around joint:

Remedy 1—Avoid hot spicy foods, spinach, and tomatoes.

Remedy 2—Coconut/castor oil pack. Pour 1 tbsp castor oil and 1 tbsp coconut oil onto a cotton cloth/facecloth and add 4 drops peppermint or lavender essential oil. Place over specific areas of pain for at least 15 minutes while lying in relaxation pose.

Remedy 3—Daily intake of curcuma (turmeric powder) by taking 1/2 tsp turmeric in warm milk or warm water twice daily.

Remedy 4—Gentle daily yoga postures after a cooling coconut oil self-massage.

For all types of arthritis: Take 1 tsp *triphala* with 1/2 cup warm water at night an hour before bed.

Acne

This skin-inflamed condition is caused by excess *pitta* in your system. This can be caused by eating a *pitta*-provoking diet (spicy, salty, oily foods, alcohol), as well as stress, intensity, hormonal changes, excess heat, or sun.

Remedy 1—Eat *pitta*-pacifying foods that are cooling and soothing in nature, such as coconut, coriander, mint, rice, oatmeal, blueberries, leafy greens, applesauce, etc.

Remedy 2—Make your own healing skin tonic by using 10 ml of rosehip oil as a carrier, add 15 drops of helichrysum essential oil, 5 drops of lemon essential oil, and 5 drops of lavender essential oil.

Remedy 3—Drink 1/4 cup aloe vera gel with 1/4 tsp turmeric powder 2 times per day half and hour before breakfast and dinner.

Remedy 4—Make a mask for your face with baking soda and water. Start with 2 tbsp of baking soda, plus 1/4 tsp of neem powder (optional) and slowly add a bit of water until you have the consistency of a paste. Gently apply the paste to your face and leave it on for 5-15 minutes before washing off with lukewarm water.

Remedy 5—A cooling breathing practice called *sheetali pranayama* is calming and cooling to the system.

Cold

When our immune system is weak, we are more susceptible to picking up germs, viruses, and bacteria. We feel weak and may have some or all of these symptoms; a runny nose, congestion, cough, aches, and pains in the body. We generally feel pretty crummy. Make sure to rest and take the time off of work to nip your cold in the bud so that it does not last as long. Avoid cold, heavy foods and all dairy. For specific symptoms of cough and congestion, see those tips as well.

Remedy 1—If you catch your cold early on, take a combination of echinacea and goldenseal. You can purchase a tincture at your local health food store.

Remedy 2—Boil 1 cup of water. Add 1/2 tsp grated ginger, 1 tsp of fresh lemon juice, pinch of cinnamon and cayenne, and 1 tsp of honey.

Remedy 3—Tulsi (holy basil). This Ayurvedic herb has many uses and is very good for supporting your body when you have a cold. Take 1 tsp of tulsi powder, mix in hot water, and drink as a tea throughout the day.

Remedy 4—*Kapalabhati pranayama*. This breathing practice heats up the body and assists in clearing obstructions.

Remedy 5—In your bath add 1/4 cup of baking soda along with 1 tsp of ginger powder.

Remedy 6—Boost your system with Vitamin C, which you can purchase at your health food store.

Congestion

Congestion, or obstruction in the body, is connected to excess *kapha*. Avoid dairy as well as cold, heavy, sugary, or oily foods, and smoking. For both sinus and chest congestion, we recommend the following remedies:

Remedy 1—*Neti* pot to cleanse the sinus cavities. Note, if the blockage in the sinuses is extreme, begin with the steam below.

Remedy 2—Steam. Get a large bowl and fill it with very hot water. Add 5 drops of tulsi or clary sage essential oils. Cover your head with a towel over the bowl and inhale deeply with your mouth open slightly.

Remedy 3—*Kapalabhati pranayama*. This breathing practice heats up the body and assists in clearing obstructions.

Constipation

Remedy 1—Drink warm water with fresh lemon first thing in the morning after tongue scraping. Do this every morning to cleanse the system.

Remedy 2—1 tsp *triphala* powder in 1/2 cup warm water before bed. Continue as long as needed.

Remedy 3—Massage the belly in a clockwise direction with warmed sesame oil at night before bed and in the morning before showering.

Remedy 4—Take 1/4 cup pure aloe vera gel in the morning half hour before breakfast. If needed continue daily for up to 3 months.

Cough

Dry cough: A dry cough is associated with excess *vata* as it has the same qualities as *vata*. Eat *vata*-pacifying foods such as warm, lightly spiced, and nourishing foods and avoid dry, cold, or light foods.

Remedy 1—Boil 1 cup of organic milk (or milk substitute) with 1/2 tsp of turmeric and 1/4 tsp of ginger powder. Drink this at night to help settle the dry, tickly, irritated feeling in the throat.

Remedy 2—Boil 1 cup of water with 1/2 tsp grated ginger. Let cool to drinking temperature and add 1/2 tsp honey.

Remedy 3—Licorice tea. There are many varieties that you can get at your health food store these days. Ideally, take 1/2 tsp of licorice powder and add to boiled water. Drink as a tea.

Mucous-y cough: When you have phlegm, it is a signal of *kapha* accumulation so avoid cold, heavy, and oily foods and favour warm, light, and spicy foods. If you see a yellow or green tinge to the mucous, *pitta* is involved and possibly some infection may be there as well.

Remedy 1—Boil 1 cup of warm water with 1/2 tsp of ginger powder and a pinch of cinnamon, nutmeg, black pepper, cloves, and cardamom. Drink this as needed.

Remedy 2—Take 1/4 tsp of black pepper and mix with 1 tsp of honey. Take this after meals.

Hangover

Remedy 1—Not drinking too much in the first place, it just feels rotten. (Seriously! Nothing like the obvious . . .)

Remedy 2—Simply continue drinking water to rehydrate yourself and flush your liver.

Remedy 3—Drink coconut water to replenish important electrolytes such as sodium, potassium, and some magnesium.

Remedy 4—CCF Tea. Take 1 tsp each of fennel seed, cumin seed, and coriander seed. Add along with 4 cups water to a small pot and bring to boil. When mixture has reached a boil, turn down to simmer for 10-15 minutes. Strain and drink. This balances the system and makes it a more alkaline environment internally.

Remedy 5—Dr. Vasant Lad of the Ayurvedic Institute recommends drinking one glass of water with 1 tsp lime juice, 1 tsp sugar, and a pinch of salt. Just before drinking, add 1/2 tsp baking soda.

Headaches

Remedy 1—Add 1 drop of peppermint essential oil and 1 drop of rosemary essential oil to palms. Rub hands together vigorously and place cupped hands over nose. Inhale deeply. Repeat until body begins to relax. You can also apply essential oils to a diffuser and allow it to infuse the space you are in.

Remedy 2—Massage neck and area of tension with a base of sesame oil (if you are a cold *vata* type) or coconut oil (if you are a hot *pitta* type) or sunflower oil (if you are a cool *kapha* type) with a few drops of rosemary and eucalyptus oil.

Remedy 3—Massage temples with vetiver or sandalwood essential oils in a base of coconut oil.

Indigestion

Before you eat anything, your digestive fire must be stoked and able to burn up whatever you choose to ingest. Otherwise, you may experience gas, bloating, heaviness, fatigue after eating, or nausea.

Remedy 1—Cut a thin slice of fresh ginger, sprinkle with rock salt, add a squeeze of lemon and eat a half hour before your meal. If this seems like too much of a hassle, at the very least drink a cup of ginger tea before your meals.

Remedy 2—Avoid eating fruit with other foods as this is a poor food combination and will tax your digestive capacity.

Remedy 3—Drink cumin/coriander/fennel tea (CCF). Take 1 tsp each of fennel seed, cumin seed, and coriander seed. Add along with 4 cups water to a small pot and bring to boil. When mixture has reached a boil, turn down to simmer for 10-15 minutes. Strain and drink.

Remedy 4—Relax before you eat and make sure you're eating sitting down in a stress-free, calm, and quiet environment.

Remedy 5—Slow down and chew your food. Seriously. This is will help you to not over-eat.

Insomnia/Sleeplessness

Remedy 1—Use a nebulizer/diffuser in your room at night with a few drops of any one of these essential oils: vetiver, geranium, lavender, clary sage, or spikenard.

Remedy 2—Drink 1/2 cup of warm organic milk (or soy milk or almond milk) with 1/4 tsp grated nutmeg (or powdered, if you don't have whole nutmeg) stirred in. Nutmeg is like the valium of the spice world. Continue for at least a week to see results.

Remedy 3—Practice *nadi shodhana pranayama* for 5-10 minutes before bed.

Remedy 4—Avoid eating at least 2-3 hours before bed as this disrupts sleep and the body cannot rest—it is too busy digesting!

Remedy 5—A guided sleep visualization (guided by you). While lying in bed with closed eyes and starting at the feet, go through each part of the body asking it to relax. Continue this practice until you have gone through the whole body. Keep doing this for at least a week and beyond, and through auto-suggestion your body and mind will slowly begin to respond.

Menstrual pain

Remedy 1—Castor oil pack. Apply 1 tbsp castor oil onto a cotton cloth or facecloth and place over pelvic area. Keep on for at least 15 minutes until pain subsides.

Remedy 2—Aromatherapy oils of geranium, lavender, chamomile, and clary sage. Apply a few drops of each to palms (you can also just use one oil and keep it simple). Rub hands together vigorously and place cupped hands over nose. Inhale deeply. Repeat until body begins to relax. You can also use essential oils in a diffuser and allow them to infuse the space you are in.

Nausea

Remedy 1—1 inch fresh ginger grated into a cup of hot water. Steep for 15 minutes, strain, and drink.

Remedy 2—Add 3 cups boiling water to a big bowl. Add two drops eucalyptus oil, one drop peppermint oil, and one drop ginger oil. Place a towel so that it covers your head and the bowl, and lean over the steaming bowl for a few minutes while inhaling and exhaling deeply. This allows for expanded breathing and relieves symptoms of nausea.

PMS

Remedy 1—Place 2 drops of geranium essential oil in your palms and inhale deeply as often as needed. Try this at least 5 days before your menses begins.

Remedy 2—Evening Primrose oil as directed by your healthcare practitioner.

Remedy 3—Take 1/4 cup of aloe vera gel two times a day, three days before your menses starts.

Remedy 4—*Nadi shodhana*—daily alternate nostril breathing practice—will help to balance your hormones and relax your mind and body. Do this morning and night.

Remedy 5—Follow a soothing, *vata*-pacifying yoga practice to balance and calm.

Rashes

Skin rashes are an expression of too much *pitta* (heat) in the body. Anything that will help you cool and calm internally and externally will be beneficial. Stay out of the sun and away from heated situations, people, or in-laws.

Remedy 1—Eat *pitta*-pacifying foods that are cooling and soothing in nature such as coconut, coriander, mint, rice, oatmeal, blueberries, leafy greens, applesauce, etc.

Remedy 2—Drink 1/4 cup aloe vera gel with 1/4 tsp turmeric powder 2 times per day.

Remedy 3—Take a bunch of fresh cilantro, chop it, and throw it in a blender with enough water to make a pulpy paste that you can apply directly on the rash.

Remedy 4—Try the cooling-breathing practice, *sheetali pranayama*, to calm the system.

Sore Throat

Remedy 1—Take 1 tsp of salt and 1/2 tsp of turmeric powder in 1 cup of hot water. Gargle at least 3 times per day.

Remedy 2—In the evening, boil 1 cup of organic milk with 1/2 tsp turmeric, 1/4 tsp licorice powder, and 1/4 tsp ginger.

Remedy 3—Stop talking. Keeping *mouna* (silence) as much as possible will help your throat heal faster.

Remedy 4—Omit any cold, dry, or scratchy foods that may aggravate your throat such as crackers, rice cakes, and cereals as well as dairy foods (other than the boiled milk suggestion above).

Remedy 5—The Humming Bee breathing practice, *bhramari pranayama*, is very soothing for the throat.

Upper Respiratory Blues: Colds, Coughs, and Sniffles

Remedy 1—Ayurvedic Cold and Cough Tea: 1 tsp turmeric, 1 lemon sliced with skins on, 1 inch ginger sliced with skin on, and a pinch black pepper. Boil 2 cups water. Add ingredients and lower to simmer for 15 minutes. Strain. Add 2-4 tsp honey. Drink warm.

Remedy 2—A nebulizer! This is a diffuser that is almost like a humidifier and releases essential oils into the air. Every home should have one as most essential oils are anti-microbial and purify the air and lungs during the cold season. Eucalyptus, tulsi (holy basil), rosemary, and wintergreen are some favourites.

Remedy 3—Add boiling water to a bowl. Add a few drops of eucalyptus, tulsi, rosemary, or wintergreen essential oils or a blend of any of these (only 2 or 3 drops in total). Put a towel over your head, and stand over the bowl allowing the steam to deliver these power-packed essential oils directly into your respiratory system so you can breathe easier. This also sends those germs packing right out of your system!

Remedy 4—Gargle! Each morning and evening take 1/4 cup warm water and add 1/2 tsp salt and 1/2 tsp turmeric. Gargle, gargle, gargle right to the back of the throat and then spit it out. Repeat until all liquid is finished.

Remedy 5—Genius Ayurvedic cough syrup: 1 cup fresh basil leaves (squeeze juice out of leaves by grinding in a mortar and pestle or extracting in a juicer), 1 inch grated and squeezed ginger juice, and 1 tbsp honey. Mix together. Slug back. Relief!

Chapter 42

Tongue and Face Diagnosis

Morning Tongue Analysis: An Ayurvedic Health Assessment Tool

Do you remember going to the doctor when you were young and they asked you to stick out your tongue? They would then use a wooden tongue depressor to look at the back of your throat (more often than not inducing the gag reflex).

Well, thank goodness we are not doing that. In Ayurveda we use the signs on the tongue as a main tool of diagnosing our current health condition. This is helpful for self-awareness and deeper observation. Some of our internal imbalances take years to develop, so give yourself and your tongue time and kindness and patience to heal.

Stick out your tongue! What do you see?

Is it coated with a milky-white layer or is it more yellowish or greyish? Do you see lines, squiggles, cracks, indents down the middle, or teeth marks on the side? These are all little clues as to what may be going on internally.

It is an excellent morning practice to look at your tongue before your tongue-scraping ritual. Do not be alarmed, just be prepared to see some healthy changes that may begin to manifest with consistent Ayurvedic lifestyle practices and habits.

The tongue is a comprehensive map of your health!

The tongue mirrors the organs of the body and can give you a clue as to what may be going on with your digestion, your immune system, and provide you with a current health analysis. A mark, discoloration and/or sensitivity of a certain part of the tongue directly reflects an imbalance in the corresponding organ. (See diagram below)

Dosha Tongue Diagnosis

A milky/chalky whitish tongue indicates a *kapha* imbalance with possible mucous and congestion, and *ama* or toxins in the respiratory system. An "oily" thick tongue may indicate excess *kapha* and high cholesterol.

A greenish or yellowish coating indicates a *pitta* imbalance with possible excess heat and inflammation and toxins in the blood and/or liver. May also show red spots or dots in specific areas on tongue, indicating inflammation.

A brownish or greyish coating indicates a *vata* imbalance with possible dryness, constipation, excess cold, and pain in the body with accumulated toxins in the colon. Small irregular cracks on the tongue may also indicate a *vata* imbalance.

Teeth imprints around the corners and sides of the tongue are signs of malabsorption of nutrients. This may be due to poor digestion, over-eating, a dry or sluggish colon, or toxins in the digestive tract. Improper food combining can also often cause indigestion and result in malabsorption. A simple remedy to balance digestion over time and cleanse the colon is by starting each day with your tongue scraping and drinking warm water with lemon.

A trembling tongue is a possible sign of fear, anxiety, stress, too much caffeine, and a compromised nervous system. These are mostly signs of a *vata* imbalance.

Your Irresistible Life

What is Your Tongue Telling You?

Signs, marks and possible coating on your tongue can tell you a lot about your current state of health. Use this simple guide to seasonally observe your tongue so you can adjust your diet, lifestyle and habits according to Ayurvedic principles and seasonal practices.

Intestines (Large and Small, Colon)
Indigestion, constipation, bloating, diarrhoea, flatulence, irritable bowel syndrome, diverticulitis, colitis, psoriasis, eczema, headaches, inability to lose weight, excess anxiety. This list goes on as good digestion, absorption and assimilation is the key to good health

Right Kidney
Excess sugar in diet, kidney stones, insufficient excercise, poor hydration, excess fear.

Spinal Column
Stress, mechanical or muscular problems, irregular posture, pinched nerve, arthritis, muscle spasm, slipped disk, tingling or weakness in spine. Neck tension, curvature of spine, headaches.

Left Kidney
Same as right kidney

Spleen
Anaemia, constipation, scanty urination, difficulty breathing, chronic cough, loss of appetite, light-headedness, lethargy, excess thinking.

Pancreas
Abdominal pain, fever, nausea, jaundice, weight loss, weakness.

Stomach
Indigestion, overeating, nausea, bloating, acid stomach, excess fear and guilt.

Liver
Congestion, toxicity, fatigue, high cholesterol, hypoglycemia, jaundice, skin conditions/diseases, excess anger.

Right Lung
Congestion, asthma, hay fever, allergies, restricted breathing, grief.

Left Lung
Congestion, restricted breathing, asthma, hay fever, allergies, grief.

Heart
Heartburn, acid reflux, high cholesterol, low immunity, mental and emotional stress, lack of love.

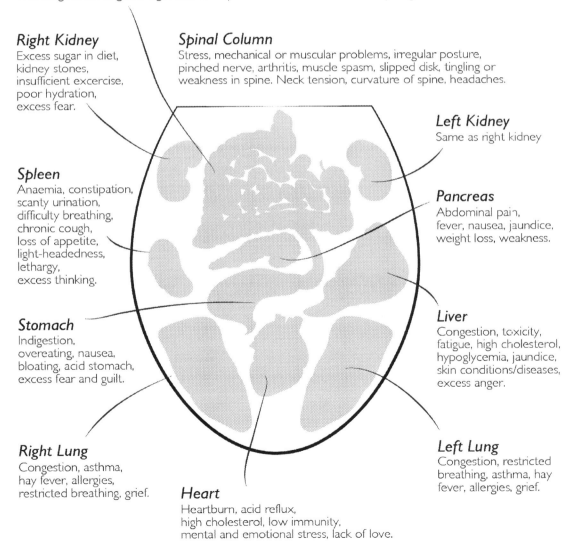

Spring
What Does Your Tongue Tell You?

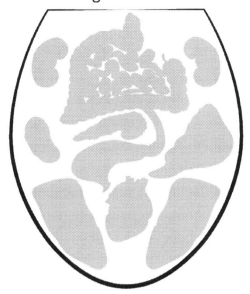

Fall
What Does Your Tongue Tell You?

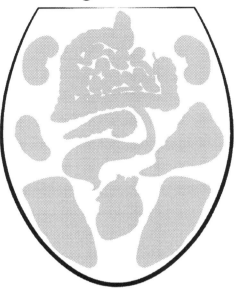

Winter
What Does Your Tongue Tell You?

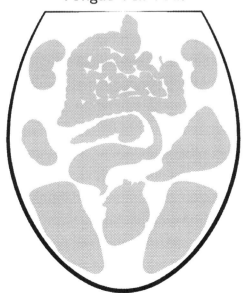

Summer
What Does Your Tongue Tell You?

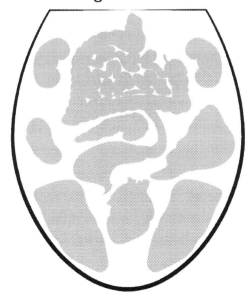

What is Your Face Reflecting?

Your face is a reflection of your thoughts and emotions. No amount of cosmetic surgery can resolve the internal state of the mind. Observing your facial lines, wrinkles, and marks you can gain an understanding of your deeper thoughts and emotions that may otherwise remain hidden and repressed or unexpressed.

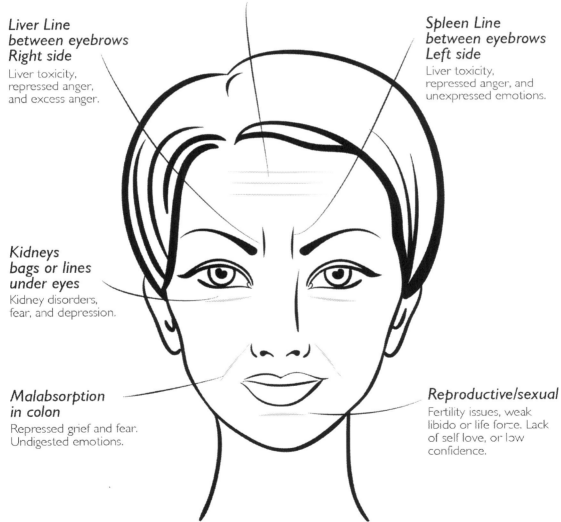

Worry Lines
Vata imbalance, anxiety, repressed nervous tension.

Liver Line between eyebrows Right side
Liver toxicity, repressed anger, and excess anger.

Spleen Line between eyebrows Left side
Liver toxicity, repressed anger, and unexpressed emotions.

Kidneys bags or lines under eyes
Kidney disorders, fear, and depression.

Malabsorption in colon
Repressed grief and fear. Undigested emotions.

Reproductive/sexual
Fertility issues, weak libido or life force. Lack of self love, or low confidence.

Chapter 43

Not So Common, Common Sense Ayurvedic Tips

TIP #1
"No ice in my drink please waiter..."

Did you know iced drinks hamper digestion and put out *agni*—the fire of digestion?

TIP #2
One *anjali*—or one of your own closely cupped handsful—is the size of your stomach and that is the portion of food that is perfect for you at each meal. When we put in more food, the stomach expands until it is full. The more you eat, the more it expands. Makes you think, doesn't it?

TIP #3
Eight glasses of water a day! How many times have you heard that? Ayurveda is not a one size fits all science of life so actually we do need to drink enough water daily, but only according to our true thirst. That measure will be true to our personal Ayurvedic body type or constitution.

TIP #4
Banana or no banana? Mixing fruit with other foods creates a fermented cocktail in the stomach and disrupts proper digestion leading to gas, bloating, and indigestion. Banana milkshakes are yummy but mixing fruit with milk is mayhem for the system. Cooked fruit is an exception as the quality and properties have changed through the cooking process. Eat your fruit alone on an empty stomach to make sure the previous meal has properly digested.

TIP #5
Cooked honey is toxic to the system. Cooked honey becomes an indigestible substance that sticks to the mucous membranes and clogs subtle channels in the body creating toxins in the system. Eat your honey raw and uncooked!

TIP #6
Turn off your computer and all electronics at least one hour before bed, dim the lights, and begin to unwind for a better night's sleep. It is scientifically proven that the lights of most electronic devices coax your brain to believe that your eyes are taking in daylight.

TIP #7
Don't eat if you are not hungry. Sounds so simple, doesn't it?

TIP #8
Not all yoga is created equal. Be sure you're not aggravating your *dosha* with your yoga practice. *Pitta* people, *get out* of those hot yoga classes!

TIP #9
Ladies, rest and relax during the first couple days of your period. No gym, no lifting weights, no extra stress, no running 10 km . . . just slow down, eat well, and rest. This will help to reduce PMS and any annoying pain associated with your period.

TIP #10
Reduce gas and bloating with ginger. Try ginger tea or even a thin slice of ginger with a squeeze of lemon and pinch of rock salt half an hour before meals to improve digestion.

TIP #11
The breath is a reflection of the mind and is connected to the nervous system. Slow down and take 10 deep, calm breaths as often as you can remember throughout the day to reduce stress and tension.

Epilogue

So much can change in a moment, a day, a week, a month, a year.

Where were you a year ago? How were you showing up in your life at that time? What looks and feels different now?

Your day-to-day recommitment to your crystallized intention is paramount for creating the life you want and deserve.

It does not matter how many times you fall off of the path. What matters is your courage and willingness to get back to the truth of what you desire and take action towards your goals. The key here is acceptance and love. No amount of blame, criticism, or judgment of yourself will get you any closer to the infinite being that you are.

You have a great purpose that is unique to you.

To fulfill your purpose you must align your heart and head. You must be as healthy as you can possibly be in body, mind, and spirit.

Through this book we have come together to share our knowledge, wisdom, current practices, and life experiences with the intention of offering options for living in alignment with Nature. It can be overwhelming and confusing these days with media sources and outlets rattling off information about new health trends and studies toting all sorts of zany ideas.

Ayurveda is not a passing trend. Ayurveda is not a flash-in-the-pan health fad. Ayurveda is as old as humankind. It is the art of living in alignment with Nature, the science of understanding your internal environment (*dosha*) and how that interacts, responds, and relates to the external environment.

Just remember: What may work for someone else may not work for you. No one is like you. Only you have your specific body, personality, mental proclivities, genetic predispositions, and *karmas*.

Use the tools and practices in this book not just for a season but let them be the foundation and building blocks for a long and joyful existence.

Thank you for joining us on this journey. We are deeply honoured.

May the spirit of Ayurveda and Yoga settle in your cells, touch your hearts yearning, and awaken the ultimate power within you.

May love and light be your guide through this ever-changing landscape of experience we call life.

With love & to your health,
Glynnis & Madhuri

Glossary

Abhyanga
An Ayurvedic massage that utilizes specific oils according to one's *dosha* to balance the nervous system, boost immunity, and strengthen the body.

Agnihotra
A traditional Vedic healing fire ceremony with the intention of cleansing and spiritually purifying the atmosphere.

Ama
Anything that is not digested (physical, mental, or emotional) creates this toxic by-product that leads to imbalance and eventually disease in the body/ mind.

Asafoetida
This spice, also commonly known as *hing,* is a dried gum oleoresin from a perennial rhizome. This pungent spice is used in cooking to enhance the flavour of food, and also as a digestive aid to reduce flatulence.

Asana
Literally means "to sit down" or "steady seat". In contemporary terminology, *asana* also refers to the physical yoga postures that one would experience during a yoga class to improve the body's flexibility and health, with the overarching outcome being to cultivate the ability to sit still in meditation for periods of time.

Chyawanprash
A jam-like formula prepared according to a specific Ayurvedic recipe with 49 herbs, spices, honey, and ghee. The base ingredient is *amla* or Indian Gooseberry which has a very high concentration of Vitamin C. This tonic is used to rejuvenate the body and boost immunity.

Dinacharya
Translates as "daily-routine". In Ayurveda this is a consistent practice aligned with the cycles of nature and observed according to one's *dosha*. In Ayurveda the daily routine is considered essential to balancing the constitution and bringing about lasting change in the body, mind, and consciousness.

Dhatus
The seven physical layers of body tissues: plasma, blood, muscle, adipose, bone, marrow, and reproductive tissue.

Dosha
Translates as "fault" or "disease". In Ayurveda, *doshas* are considered to be the pathogenic factors that cause disease. An imbalance of any of the three biological humors: *vata*, *pitta*, or *kapha* cause imbalance and disease. These three energetic principles are uniquely expressed in various proportions in every individual and are referred to as "your Ayurvedic constitution".

Ghee
Ghee is simply clarified butter. Unsalted butter is boiled at a low temperature until the moisture has evaporated and the milk solids and oil has separated. The oil is stored in a glass jar and solidifies at room temperature, remaining unspoiled outside of refrigeration. Ghee is considered a purifying food in Ayurveda, bringing harmony to body and mind, also acting as a vehicle for herbs and medicines to the deeper tissues.

Havan
A sacred fire ceremony for purification where there is an invocation of positive energies, recitation of *mantras* or prayers, and offerings made to the fire.

Homa
See "Havan".

Kapha
Kapha is one of the three *doshas*. It is comprised of water and earth and governs structure, lubrication, anabolic activity, and fluids in the body.

Kombu
This is a type of seaweed/sea vegetable that refers to any type of edible kelp.

Masala
A *masala* is a combination of several different spices and/or herbs mixed or blended together.

Nadi
Translates as "river" or "flow". One's *pranic*/subtle body is comprised of thousands of these energetic channels that weave in and out of the various chakras. In Yoga, we focus on three main *nadis*: *ida*, *pingala*, and *sushumna* that carry vital energy through the body.

Nasya
One of the five purification techniques in "*panchakarma*" where medicated oil drops are inhaled through the nostrils.

Neti (Jala Neti)
One of yoga's *"shatkarma"* cleansing practices that involves pouring saline water through the nasal passages. This is very good for helping to clear: mucous, common colds, allergies, cloudy/ dull mind, depression, sore throat, sinusitis, and other ailments.

Neem
This herb comes from the evergreen neem tree and is dried into a powder to be used as a tea, added into a herbal formula, or applied as a topical medicine. An excellent remedy to cool, clear, and purify irritated and inflamed skin. Working as both an antiseptic and anti-inflammatory, neem is a specific tonic for the *pitta dosha*.

Oil pulling
This is a traditional Ayurvedic practice of swishing oil around the gums and teeth for 10-20 minutes first thing in the morning so that toxins and bacteria are "pulled" into the oil and then released out of the mouth. About a tablespoon of either sesame, sunflower, or coconut oil is used depending on the constitution.

Ojas
A subtle substance that is the end result of properly digested food. *Ojas* literally translates as "vigor" and is the essence of our stamina, immunity, clarity, and enthusiasm for life.

Panchamahabhutas
The five great elements that make up all of creation: earth, water, fire, air, and ether.

Pancha Karma
An ancient practice of five actions of purification and detoxification including: emesis, purgation, enema, *nasya*, and blood letting.

Prabha
This is a Sanskrit word meaning "the light", "light" or "dawns first light" or "luminosity".

Prakruti
One's original or true nature: The Ayurvedic blueprint of an individual that is established at conception and remains unaltered throughout the life. The unique proportions of *vata*, *pitta*, and *kapha* for an individual (the Ayurvedic constitution).

Prana
The vital energy or life force that animates the body and all things.

Pitta
One of the three *doshas*. *Pitta* is composed of fire and water and governs transformation, metabolic function, and biochemical activity.

Rishis
The *rishis* were the sages, seers, or scribes of the spiritual science of the *Vedas*, culling the knowledge from Nature's secrets and the great wisdom of the Universe.

Savasana
The final posture in a yoga class, known as "corpse pose". The entire body relaxes on the floor in a supine position with feet apart and arms out to the sides of the body. This *asana* integrates all of the experiences from the yoga class and brings about a sense of deep relaxation.

Sadhana
A daily discipline or practice imbued with a spiritual intention to cultivate and expand awareness.

Sneha
This is a Sanskrit word used both for affection, love, and friendship and also as an Ayurvedic term for oleation and other therapies where oil is applied internally or externally. The connection can be made to self-love through the Ayurvedic daily practice of massaging the body with oil.

Tahini
An oily, creamy paste made from ground, hulled sesame seeds.

Tridosha
The combination of the three biological humors or principles known in Ayurveda as *vata*, *pitta*, and *kapha*.

Triphala
An ancient Ayurvedic formula composed of three fruits; *amalaki*, *bibhitaki* and *haritaki*. This formula has all of the six tastes and is balancing for all three *doshas*.

Tulsi
Known in Ayurveda as the "Queen of herbs" and also known as "Holy Basil". This versatile healing herb is used as the dried leaf in teas or the powdered herb in formulas. Tulsi has been classified as an adaptogenic herb that is used as a restorative tonic to support the immune system and promote wellness.

Vikruti
The current state of physical, mental, and emotional health in relation to the *prakruti*, original nature.

Vata
One of the three Ayurvedic *doshas*. Air and ether make up *vata dosha*, also known as "*vayu*" or "wind". *Vata* governs movement, kinetic energy, the nervous system, and circulation.

Bibliography

Lad, V. (1998). *The Complete Book of Ayurvedic Home Remedies.* New York: Three Rivers Press.

Miller, Dr. L. (1995). *Ayurveda & Aromatherapy. The Earth Essential Guide to Ancient Wisdom and Modern Healing.* Wisconsin: Lotus Press.

Raichur, P. (1997). *Absolute Beauty. Radiant Skin and Inner Harmony through the ancient secrets of Ayurveda.* New York: Harper Collins

Saraswati, Swami, S. (1969) *Asana Pranayama Mudra Bandha.* Bihar: Bihar School of Yoga

Sondhi, Amrita. (2006). *The Modern Ayurvedic Cookbook: Healthful, Healing Recipes for Life.* Vancouver: Arsenal Pulp Press

Tiwari, M. (1995) *Ayurveda, Secrets of Healing.* Wisconsin: Lotus Press

Tiwari, M. (1995) *Ayurveda, A Life of Balance.* Vermont: Healing Arts Press

Yarema, M.D. T., Rhoda, D., Brannigan, J. (2006) *Eat. Taste. Heal An Ayurvedic Guidebook and Cookbook for Modern Living.* Hawaii: Five Elements Press

Resources

Aromatherapy

Floracopeia
www.floracopeia.com

The Mystic Masala Ayurvedic Aromatherapy
www.themysticmasala.com

Ayurvedic Centres and Inspiration

Glynnis & Madhuri
www.glynnisandmadhuri.com

Dr. Claudia Welch
www.drclaudiawelch.com

John Douillard's LifeSpa
www.lifespa.com

Madhuri Ayurveda & Yoga
www.madhuriayurvedayoga.com

Mount Madonna Institute
www.mountmadonnainstitute.org

Rasa Ayurveda
www.rasaayurveda.com

The Ayurvedic Institute
www.ayurveda.com

The Chopra Centre
www.chopra.com

The Wise Earth School
www.wiseearth.com

Ayurvedic Cookbooks

Eat-Taste-Heal: An Ayurvedic Cookbook for Modern Living
Dr. Thomas Yarema M.D., Daniel Rhoda, Chef Johnny Brannigan

The Modern Ayurvedic Cookbook: Healthful, Healing Recipes for Life
Amrita Sondhi

The Ayurvedic Cookbook: Vegetarian Recipes for Body, Mind and Spirit
Ginna Bell Bragg, David Simon

Ayurvedic Cooking for Self-Healing
Usha Lad, Vasant Lad

Ayurveda: A Life of Balance—The Complete Guide to Ayurvedic Nutrition & Body Types with Recipes
Maya Tiwari

Ayurvedic Herbs & Products

Banyan Botanicals
www.banyanbotanicals.com

Madhuri Ayurveda & Yoga
www.madhuriayurvedayoga.com

The Mystic Masala Ayurvedic Aromatherapy
www.themysticmasala.com

Index

A

Abhyanga 21, 25, 208, 233
Achy joints 215
Acne 15–16, 18, 100, 127, 216
Affirmations 5
Agni 48, 87, 100, 124, 180, 228
Agnihotra 124, 233
Air 11, 14, 26, 30, 41, 47, 53, 57, 60, 75, 93, 99, 100, 106, 121, 123, 133, 137, 139, 167, 180, 222, 235, 237
Almonds 31, 64, 128, 143, 183, 185, 189, 208–209
Aloe vera 62, 101, 111, 128–129, 216, 218, 221
Ama 47–50, 81, 87, 167, 214, 223, 233
Anjali 228
Anxiety 16, 18, 96, 139, 152, 159, 226
Aromatherapy 23, 72–73, 112, 114, 138, 150, 151, 178, 191–192, 208, 220, 237, 239, 245
Arthritis 216
Asafoetida 63, 67, 88, 142, 147, 233
Asana 38, 201, 233, 236–237
Ayana 207

B

Beauty v, xxi, 7, 13, 20, 35, 37, 44, 55, 59, 69, 70, 85, 96, 110, 151, 153–154, 163, 188, 194, 201, 237, 245
Bhramari pranayama 222
Bloating 16, 18, 48–49, 90, 173, 179, 219, 228–229

C

Cardamom 30, 60, 63, 68, 73, 88, 102, 107, 138, 142–143, 146, 151–152, 168, 178, 180, 182–183, 186–188, 192, 209, 211, 218
Castor oil 215, 220
Cat stretch 156
Ceremony 45, 69, 84–85, 124–126, 163–165, 204, 206, 233–234
Chai 55, 143, 183, 186
Chickpeas 63, 102, 104, 142, 181–182, 185–186
Child's Pose 156
Chin mudra 203
Cilantro 15, 30, 61–62, 67–68, 89, 102, 105, 128–129, 147, 186, 221
Clary sage 71, 73, 150–151, 178, 191, 192, 217, 220
Cleanse 30, 47–50, 60–61, 70, 81, 85, 87–90, 93, 110, 117, 127–130, 133, 138, 146, 149, 167–169, 173, 189, 213–214, 217, 224, 245
Coconut oil 23, 97–98, 109, 111, 127, 128, 215–216, 219, 235
Colitis 16
Colon 14, 138, 224
Congestion 16, 59–62, 68, 74, 81, 87, 99–100, 178, 180, 213–214, 216–217, 223
Constipation 16, 18, 48, 90, 173, 217, 224
Constitution 12, 14, 17, 27, 31, 47, 49, 139, 146, 228, 233–235
Coriander 30, 63–64, 67, 88, 98, 101–103, 128, 142–143, 145–147, 152, 168, 182–183, 185–186, 216, 218–219, 221
Corpse pose 236
Creativity xxi, 4, 7, 18, 41, 44, 74, 126

D

Dairy 30, 60, 62, 64, 88, 89, 103, 129, 143, 168–169, 181, 183, 216–217, 222
Dates 102–103, 107, 141–143, 182, 187, 209
Depression 188, 193, 213, 235
Dhatus 48, 50, 188, 234
Diagnosis 12, 223, 228
Diet 15–17, 19, 26–27, 50, 61–62, 82, 87, 89, 101, 127, 130, 139–140, 146, 167, 169, 181, 216
Dinacharya 20, 233

E

Earth xv, xix, xxi, 11, 14, 15, 26–28, 30–31, 45, 61, 87, 180–181, 206, 234–235, 237, 240, 245
Echinacea 64, 217
Epsom salts 23, 25, 150, 191
Essential oils 23, 60, 71–74, 98, 111–113, 150–152, 178, 191–192, 208, 213, 217, 219–220, 222

Ether 11, 14–16, 26, 30, 56, 139, 167, 180, 235, 237
Eucalyptus 60, 73–74, 112, 138, 178, 191–193, 208, 213, 219–220, 222
Evening Primrose oil 221

F

Face diagnosis 223, 228
Fall food 139, 142–145, 169
Fall yoga 138, 154, 168
Fatigue 12, 16, 48, 135, 219
Fertility 84
Fire v, 11, 14, 15, 26, 30, 45, 48, 76, 87, 93, 98, 100–101, 110–111, 124–126, 140, 146, 167, 177–178, 180–181, 219, 228, 233–236
Food prayer 32
Frankincense xx, 191–192

G

Geranium 98, 111–112, 138, 150–152, 178, 192, 213, 220–221
Ghee 27, 30, 47, 64, 67, 87–88, 98, 101, 103, 105, 140, 143–147, 167, 168, 181, 183, 186, 209, 214, 233–234
Ginger 30, 59, 60, 62–63, 66–68, 71–73, 88, 101–102, 107, 142–143, 145–147, 151–152, 168, 178, 180–183, 184–187, 189, 191–193, 209, 215, 217–220, 222–223, 229
Goldenseal 217

H

Halitosis 16, 214
Headaches 213–214, 219
Heartburn 15–16, 100
Herbal tea 22–23, 68, 88, 128–129, 168, 208
Hindu 45, 56, 84
Homa 234
Honey 64, 68, 103, 143, 148, 174, 181, 183, 185–186, 188–190, 209, 217–218, 222, 228–229, 233

I

I Ching 205–206
Ida 81, 234

Immunity 26, 77, 81, 87, 122, 167, 177, 180–181, 188, 191, 204, 207, 214, 233, 235
India xv, xix, 11–12, 36, 50, 55, 84, 114, 124, 246
Indigestion 48, 90, 171, 179, 219, 224, 228
Inflammation 30, 100–101, 127, 224
Insomnia 16, 18, 139, 201, 214, 220
Intention 3, 5–8, 7, 25, 34, 45, 47, 49, 62, 86, 101, 124, 126, 163–166, 175, 206, 231, 233, 236

J

Jala neti 213, 235
Journals 55, 74, 95, 113, 134, 152, 174, 193

K

Kapalbhati 81
Kichari 23, 25, 66–68, 87, 89, 96, 146–147, 167, 169
Kombu 140, 234

L

Laughing meditation 123
Lavender 25, 60, 70–71, 73, 98, 101, 111–112, 138–139, 151, 190, 192, 208, 213, 216, 220
Liver 16, 30, 61, 72, 87, 101, 109, 117, 127, 200, 218, 224
Lung 61, 68–69, 81, 100, 160, 175, 181, 188, 190–191, 200, 222

M

Mandala 85–86, 126, 206
Mantra xx–xxi, 37, 45, 100, 114, 162–163, 194, 234
Masala 27, 145, 147, 234, 239, 245
Meditation 5, 19, 22, 25, 27, 34, 43, 44, 76, 82–84, 88, 105, 116, 122–123, 129, 134, 136, 154, 160, 162, 168, 194–195, 202, 233
Menstrual pain 220
Metabolism 14, 30, 178, 188
Mineral broth 22, 68, 88, 144, 149
Moisturizer 71, 106, 111, 150, 190
Mouna 36, 222
Mucous 30, 47, 53, 61, 81, 87–88, 101, 181, 213–214, 218, 223, 228, 235
Mudra 159–160, 162, 203, 237

Mung beans 63, 66–68, 87–88, 102, 142, 146, 167–168, 181–182

N

Nadi shodhana 16, 159–160, 220–221
Nasagra mudra 159–160
Nausea 16, 219–221
Neem 128–129, 216, 235
Neroli 98, 112, 138, 150–152
Neti pot 213, 217

O

Oats 63–64, 140, 142, 149, 182, 184–185, 209
Oil pulling 21, 97, 138, 178, 214, 235
Ojas 47, 140, 188, 189, 204, 207, 235
Over-eating 16, 22, 24, 26, 60, 89, 99, 140, 169, 179, 224

P

Pancha karma 49–50, 85, 235, 246
Panchamahabutas 26
Pingala 81, 234
Prabha xxi, 235
Prakruti 14, 17–19, 235–236
Prana xv, 31, 39, 41–42, 48, 81, 116, 159, 202, 235
Pranam mudra 162, 203
Pranayama 16–17, 21, 41–42, 60, 76, 81, 88, 98, 116, 121, 129, 138, 154, 159, 168, 178, 195, 201–202, 208, 216–217, 220–222, 237

Q

Quinoa 30, 61, 63–65, 89, 102, 142, 169, 182

R

Rashes 16, 100–101, 127, 221
Remedies 215, 217, 237
Rishis xv, xx, 41, 236
Ritual 20–21, 31–32, 35, 45–46, 59, 70–71, 84–86, 97, 100, 111, 124–126, 138, 149, 163–166, 178, 190, 204, 206, 223
Ritucharya 20

Routine 4, 12, 16, 20–21, 35, 56, 59, 76, 96, 100, 116, 134–135, 137, 139, 148–149, 154, 174, 177, 189, 195, 233
Rumi 137

S

Sadhana xv, xxi, 33–34, 39, 148, 236
Saffron 30, 63, 101–102, 104, 107–109, 142, 182, 186, 211
Sandalwood 60, 73, 98, 111–112, 138, 151, 219
Savasana 236
Sea salt 30, 66–67, 71, 88, 145, 147, 150, 168, 185, 191
Sesame oil 16, 21, 23, 138, 145, 149–150, 168, 178, 181, 191, 208–209, 215, 218–219
Sheetali 16, 121, 216, 221
Six tastes 28–30, 65, 104, 139–140, 144–145, 180, 184, 236
Small intestine 14, 32, 116
Sneha 139, 236
Snehana 21
So-hum 162
Solstice 124–125, 204–205
Spirulina 64, 107, 128–129
Spleen 200
Spring food 61–65, 88–89
Spring yoga 60, 76, 88
Stomach 14, 16, 49, 228
Summer food 100–104, 101–104, 130
Summer yoga 98, 116, 128
Sunflower oil 23, 60, 71, 88, 128–129, 219
Sun salutation 76
Surya namaskara 76–77, 81

T

Thirst 18, 30, 53, 228
Tofu 63, 66, 102, 142, 182
Tongue diagnosis 223, 228
Tongue scraping 214, 217, 224
Tonic 62, 68, 70, 72, 101, 106, 109, 140, 147–148, 181, 187–189, 216, 233, 235–236
Toxicity 47, 49–50, 53, 174
Tridoshic 146, 169
Triphala 88, 90, 128, 168, 170, 216–217, 236
Tulsi 143, 168, 183, 217, 222, 236

Turmeric 30, 63, 108–109, 128, 142, 168, 178, 180–182, 184–186, 215–216, 218, 221–222

U

Ujjayi 76, 195, 201–202

V

Vedas 124, 236
Vedic xxi, 45, 55, 110, 233
Vetiver 98, 112, 138, 151, 219–220
Vikruti 14, 17–19, 236
Visualization 70, 202, 204, 220

W

Water 8, 11, 14, 15, 21, 25–26, 30, 41, 47–48, 53, 59, 61, 64–68, 71–72, 74–75, 84, 87–88, 98, 100–107, 109–113, 128–129, 138, 141, 143, 145–147, 149–150, 152, 168, 178, 180–181, 183–187, 190–192, 208, 213–222, 224, 228, 234–236
Winter food 180–184, 208
Winter yoga 178, 195, 208

About the Authors

About Glynnis and Madhuri

We have both been inspired, dedicated, and successful in our individual practices and careers in the healing arts. Through our deep friendship and mutual love of Ayurveda and our desire to evolve and help others reach their highest potential—we offer powerful, life-changing experiences. We passionately apply our vibrant, authentic, and transformational teaching methods when leading our Retreats, Workshops, and on-line Seasonal Cleanses.

Our vision is to inspire you to an irresistible life where you can thrive and feel healthier, happier, and more alive than you ever thought possible.

www.glynnisandmadhuri.com

About Glynnis Osher

Glynnis (BFA, CAP) is an inspiring teacher, healer, author, artist, and visionary entrepreneur in the arts of Ayurveda and aromatherapy. She is affectionately known as "The Spice Mistress" for sharing her innovative creations in the arena of Ayurvedic aromatherapy and aroma-nutrition.

Glynnis was born and raised in South Africa where she began her career as an art director in the advertising world. She immigrated to New York in her early 20's where she was later drawn to the healing arts of Ayurveda.

Glynnis graduated from Bastyr University's AYU Academy as well as from the Wise Earth School of Ayurveda. She also received certification with the London School of Champissage, later deepening her Indian Head massage practice with *marma* training at The Ayurvedic Institute of New Mexico.

Glynnis is founder and CEO of *The Mystic Masala Ayurvedic Aromatherapy* where she is committed to social and environmental responsibility and integrity in the development of her Ayurvedic product line.

Through the daily wisdom and beauty of Ayurveda and aromatherapy, Glynnis inspires her students and clients to discover their own unique healing path where they can truly thrive in all areas of life.

www.themysticmasala.com

About Madhuri (Melanie Phillips)

Madhuri (BFA, E-RYT, CAS) is a healer, visionary, yoga teacher trainer, author, speaker, and radio host. Madhuri is an internationally known yoga teacher, certified Clinical Ayurvedic Specialist and Pancha Karma Specialist, receiving certification from the California College of Ayurveda and the Bihar School of Yoga, India, as well as advanced study with Dr. Vasant Lad.

She has received initiation as a Reiki Master and is a certified Bio-Energy Practitioner and Trainer.

Through her own seven year illness and un-diagnosable health challenges Madhuri decided to take her healing into her own hands, study Ayurveda and assist others with this wisdom to transform their health and wellbeing.

She uses the tools of Ayurveda, Yoga, and Bio-Energy Healing to help clients discover the root cause of their imbalance or disease and empower them with the wisdom and practices to live a life full of increased vitality, joy, peace, and fabulous health.

Madhuri provides transformative teachings through Yoga Teacher Training programs, on-line courses, workshops, her Ayurvedic Yoga DVD, and international retreats.

www.madhuriayurvedayoga.com